Praise for *Your Second Prime*

"Gretchen Terry-Leonard has done it! She has transformed the negative feelings and societal narrative of aging and gives the power back to the reader to enjoy this powerful phase of life. She elegantly combines science and personal anecdotes, describing the principles of healthy aging as inclusive in mind, body, and spirit—recognizing that not just one aspect is important, but investing in all is vital for experiencing joy and vitality. This book is a must read for all, helping change societal bias and the reader to find their joy. My takeaway was one of grace, acceptance, power, strength, and finding your sparkle in your Second Prime. Absolutely beautiful!"

—Amy Sullivan, PsyD, psychologist, Cleveland Clinic

"Motivating and challenging in ways I hadn't anticipated, *Your Second Prime* made me pause with intention. Every chapter felt purposeful and meaningful, guiding me deeper into understanding and exploring my own purpose in life."

—Jade Figueiredo, client president, Carat

"Inspiring, witty, science-backed, and refreshingly practical, *Your Second Prime* is the joyful roadmap to making the rest of your life the very best. Gretchen Terry-Leonard shows us all how to dream boldly, live purposefully, and embrace our next chapter with laughter and heart."

—Lindsay Harrer, US head of medical strategic engagement & partnerships, EMD Serono, Inc.

"In *Your Second Prime*, Gretchen Terry-Leonard reminds us that purpose isn't reserved for the young—it's the key to making this next chapter the most powerful one yet.

Far from a tired self-help guide or another ode to "anti-aging," *Your Second Prime* is a smart, candid, and empowering exploration of what it really means to grow older in a world obsessed with youth. With equal parts research, personal reflection, and cultural critique,

Your Second Prime inspires readers to take ownership of their aging experience. It doesn't just ask us to age gracefully, it dares us to age boldly. The real-life challenges at the end of each chapter help you live your Second Prime with purpose."
—Yolanda Newton

"Intriguing, captivating, and compelling!

Gretchen Terry-Leonard shares knowledge and expertise, along with proven scientific data to offer a new perspective for society at large. She challenges us to begin a new, more fulfilling chapter in life rather than start a period of decline in our Second Prime. Gretchen's laser-focus ability to achieve breakthroughs in our thinking is not only knowledge based, but put into practice, which she generously shares by way of challenges and habit-forming suggestions throughout the book.

She offers wisdom to embolden us to use our life experiences to add value that will stand the test of time. In short, she teaches us that it is our privilege and honor to find unmet needs that will serve society, as well as reframe how we present ourselves to the world and create a new life."
—Sandra Vila, entrepreneur, founder Sandra Vila Design House

"Too often we are on autopilot and don't take the time to stop and course correct. *Your Second Prime* is a true masterpiece for anyone who is willing to be honest with themselves and really look at what they want their life to look like. I love the continued theme and importance of living as your true, authentic self; and if you aren't, your body will tell you.

Thank you, Gretchen Terry-Leonard for sharing your wisdom backed by science and for being a catalyst for change!"
—Jenna Hall, EVP, head of enterprise sales, Rightway

"*Your Second Prime* is not just a reframe of aging; it is a timeline correction and a sacred invitation to reclaim our genius and a new chapter for regenerative living.

Gretchen Terry-Leonard's work is a powerful and timely reminder that maturity is not decline, and that you are not running out of time. You are ripening into the moment that was always meant for you. Your vitality and purpose are not bound by age, but awakened by alignment.

Her message is not only essential for those of us walking this threshold; it is also imperative for the generations watching us. The way we choose to live now becomes the blueprint for what is possible next. And her voice is a luminous guide for all of us charting that path forward."

—Lee Ann Del Carpio, founder, Deeply Human Leading Lab and Limitless Actualization

YOUR SECOND PRIME

YOUR SECOND
PRIME

DOES AGING SUCK,
OR DO WE SUCK
AT AGING?

Gretchen Terry-Leonard

HUDSON PARK PRESS

ESTABLISHED 2025 · NEWPORT BEACH, CA

Hudson Park Press
Newport Beach, CA

Library of Congress Control Number: 2025915002
Paperback ISBN: 979-8-9988365-0-3
Hardcover ISBN: 979-8-9988365-1-0
eBook ISBN: 979-8-9988365-2-7

Cover art by Jessica Riester (jrubydesigns.com)
Book cover and interior design by Christina Thiele
Editorial production by KN Literary Arts

To my husband, Lance, and our miracle, Hudson.

Contents

Introduction: Bloody Marys Do Serve a Purpose   1

1. Time Crimes: A Not-So-Pretty History of Our Aging
   Attitudes   9

2. Inconvenient Dreams: The Messengers We Try to Ignore   19

3. Beyond the Map: When Purpose Becomes Your North Star   29

4. The Midlife "Crisis": And Why It Is Really an Invitation   39

5. The Future You: An Inside Job   49

6. The Biology of Authenticity: Your Cells Know When
   You're Lying to Yourself   59

7. The Chemistry of Calm: From Hippie Wisdom to
   Harvard Research   73

8. Softening into Strength: The Science of Emotional Mastery   87

9. Wired to Connect: From Mirror Neurons
   to Belly Laughs   101

10. The Currency of Compound Experience: Investing in
    Your Second Prime   111

11. From Target Market to Market Maker: Flipping the
    Script on Aging Narratives   131

12. Beyond X and Y: Reimagining Biological Differences
    in Our Second Prime   143

13. Pretty Rebellious: The Revolution Against
    Age-Based Beauty   155

14. The Power of Three: Autonomy, Agency, and the Art
    of Optimistic Living   169

15. Your Inner Pharmacy: Harnessing Microbiome Magic   181

16. Glimmers and Wisdom: The Gift of Enhanced Joy!   201

Conclusion: Purpose, Power, and Possibility   213

References   219

Acknowledgments   245

About the Author   247

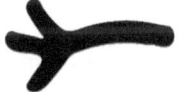

Introduction: Bloody Marys Do Serve a Purpose

About fifteen years ago a seed was planted during a lively brunch with friends in Seattle. Amid drinks adorned with umbrellas and celery stalks, we indulged in animated discussions about our future goals and dreams. The air buzzed with excitement, and for a moment our ambitions seemed limitless. As the conversation progressed, we entertained grand, outlandish plans for our future selves. But as with most discussions that dance between aspiration and reality, practicality quickly deflated our dreams. One friend's fantasy of opening a bar and restaurant was met with a grim statistic—food service has the highest failure rate. The dream was extinguished almost as soon as the words flew out of her mouth.

Yet something remarkable happened during that conversation. We began to playfully attach the word *inconvenient* to our most cherished dreams. It was a clever, irreverent way to acknowledge the boldness of our ambitions while simultaneously giving them room to breathe. *Inconvenient dreams* didn't need to follow the rules. This newly minted wordplay became the shift we needed—a way to describe those deeper, more profound desires that we often bury beneath the sensibilities of everyday life. Also, it was safer to talk tall about grandiose ideas without having imposter syndrome kick in and crush our creativity. There was no expectation that these dreams would ever see the light of day. We stopped shooting them down with harsh realities and instead began lifting them with the possibility that they could, in fact, work. Perhaps it was because everyone loves an underdog, and an inconvenient dream embodies that spirit—almost no chance of success, yet compelling in its audacity. We found ourselves rooting for these inconvenient dreams because they came from a place far more profound than the part of us that writes business plans.

The term *inconvenient dream* evolved into more than just a playful expression; it became a symbol of our collective yearning to break free from the rigid structures of our lives. In a world dominated by deadlines, expectations, and the approval of others, an inconvenient dream offers something refreshingly different. Timelines don't confine it, nor do society's judgments shape it. These dreams don't need to be genius ideas or instant successes, they are about contribution, purpose, and impact. These dreams emerge from within yourself, driven by an intrinsic desire to explore what truly matters to you. An inconvenient dream defies the conventional wisdom that your ambitions must fit neatly into the compartments of a busy life. It allows for freedom—a space where you can dream without the constraints of practicality, where your aspirations need not be justified or rationalized to anyone but yourself. Essentially, we created a new permission structure that allowed for imagination beyond a traditional goal.

That get-together was more than just a boozy brunch. It was the moment that ignited a fire within me—a determination to do more than exist as a corporate worker, to find a way to be aligned so that each day didn't feel like a grind but rather a calling. I wanted to make an impact, to chase a dream not defined by conventional success but by the value it brought to my life and the lives of others. The term *inconvenient dream* became my guiding star, urging me to dig deeper and confront the uneasy desire that I wanted to make the world a better place . . . but how?

In retrospect, I realize that the inconvenient dream concept is not unique to me; it is a universal experience. Millions of us navigate life with this inner conflict, feeling like mere cogs in the wheel when we yearn to be linchpins—creators of something meaningful. Over the centuries, countless works of art, literature, and thought have been devoted to this singular aspiration: to uncover our true purpose. I've come to understand that each of us possesses valuable gifts the world needs, and it is our responsibility to embark on the often arduous journey of discovering, manifesting, and sharing these gifts in service to ourselves and others.

My inconvenient dream was like an elusive shadow for many years—just out of reach, frustratingly shapeless and nameless. It was a persistent yet vague longing, a desire to be relevant with no clear direction. I wanted to do something meaningful that mattered, but the fog of uncertainty obscured the path. The weight of that fog was heavy. Yet, inconvenient as it was, this dream was dogged and had a stubborn streak; it clung to me, gnawing at my conscience like a relentless woodpecker—*tap, tap, tap!*

Then came the wake-up call, the moment when life grabbed me by the shoulders and gave me a good shake. Around the same time as that fateful brunch, I had a medical scare that took me from cruising on autopilot to an abrupt halt. It was one of those life-defining moments, as if the universe were holding up a giant neon sign that read: "Life is finite. Wake up!" It forced me to stop and take stock of what mattered. In all its terrifying glory, "the scare" was a gift—a moment of clarity wrapped in fear.

The words hit me like a brick. I was stunned, immobilized by the weight of the neurologist's comments. My ears began to buzz, drowning out the rest of the doctor's speech as I grappled with the sudden gravity of the situation. The room spun around me, a disorienting blur of fear and uncertainty. Even now, more than two decades later, the memory of that moment remains vivid, etched into my consciousness like a tattoo of fear and foreboding.

"When I see a woman in the prime of her life with the symptoms you have, it's usually either MS or lupus."

Extreme anxiety spread over me as I heard those words. My

solar plexus tightened in a defensive reaction, and I swallowed hard, my mouth suddenly dry. Everything I had planned for my life felt as though it was crumbling. Sitting in that cold, sterile doctor's office, the words *multiple sclerosis* and *lupus* hung in the air like a dark cloud. It was a moment that shook me to my core, a crossroads where everything I thought I knew about my body and my future was suddenly thrown into question. My fear was palpable, the confusion overwhelming, and the "what ifs" ran wild through my mind. Will I end up in a wheelchair? Will I be able to have a family, keep my marriage, sustain my career? Even as these fears tore through my thoughts, one comment struck me to the core.

The phrase "prime of her life" resonated with a chilling intensity, its implications sinking deep into my psyche. It was as if the neurologist had drawn a line in the sand, marking the boundary between youth and decline with ruthless precision. The message was clear: the prime of your life is a fleeting moment, a precious commodity not to be squandered or taken for granted. I couldn't shake it. It seemed almost cruelly ironic—how could I be in my prime when my body felt like it was betraying me? The idea of "prime" had always been tied to youth, vitality, and a sense of invincibility. But as I walked out of the clinic, something in me began to shift.

Those three little words—*prime of life*—spoken in a moment of uncertainty, became the catalyst for a profound reflection on aging and, ultimately, the inspiration for this book.

For months, while standing in line or during any idle moment, my mind would wander back to his words—*prime, prime, prime*. I replayed the conversation over and over, and what initially felt like a blow began to morph into something else. It wasn't just the fear of illness that dominated my thoughts anymore; it was the concept of time, the idea of *prime* itself. If this time in my life was supposed to be the peak, what would that mean for the years ahead?

Was it all downhill from here? Those questions haunted me but also ignited a fire within—a desire to create meaningful change. I wanted to redefine what it meant to be in my prime. The fear that had gripped me was transforming into a determination to shape a new narrative on aging.

As I began to explore this newfound awareness, my once-nebulous dream started to take shape. It wasn't an instant revelation but more like an evolution—a gradual unfolding of understanding. I stumbled, chased ideas, failed, got back up, and kept experimenting while nurturing the seed planted during that unforgettable brunch. Little by little, that tiny seed began to sprout, blossoming into something real and tangible.

I'm relieved to share that after two exhausting and frightening years of wading through differential diagnoses, the doctor's initial fears were proven incorrect—I did not have MS or lupus. The moment I received the all-clear was one of immense gratitude and overwhelming relief, a reprieve from the shadow of fear that had loomed over my life. But this experience left me with a more profound revelation that would redefine my perspective and approach to aging.

As you'll discover in the pages ahead, we are not confined to a single prime in our lives. We have the capacity for multiple primes, each offering unique opportunities for growth, fulfillment, and joy. This shift in thinking invites us to embrace the full spectrum of our existence, to redefine what it means to age with purpose and soulful beauty. The time has come for an innovative approach to living and growing older—one that celebrates the richness of experience, the wisdom gained over the years, and the boundless potential within each of us.

That seed has now grown into a visionary tree, with branches reaching out to tackle a question we all face sooner or later: How can we improve our attitudes and approach to aging? How do you live the life you want in the way you want? To put it plainly—does aging suck, or do we suck at aging? Could we, perhaps, disrupt these insidious systems and beliefs that toss people aside once they reach a certain age?

This question became the heart of what I would eventually call your Second Prime philosophy—a bold, perhaps audacious stance that challenges the prevailing narrative of decline and decay. I began to see the years ahead not as a slow descent but as a potential Second Prime—or even Third Prime—a time to harness and employ all the knowledge, skills, and strengths accumulated over the years. What if aging was an opportunity instead of a sentence? What if it was a chance for continued growth, contribution, freedom, and even reinvention? With this realization, I set out on a mission to redefine and disrupt the shame and negativity that so often go with aging, one inconvenient dream at a time.

The philosophy of *Your Second Prime* is anchored in a powerful truth—one that defies the status quo and challenges our most basic assumptions about aging. Ageism is not simply wrong; it diminishes the potential of individuals and society alike. By sidelining ourselves and others as we grow older, we do a disservice to ourselves and the world. This truth is not merely personal; it's a societal imperative, urging us to rethink how we view aging and to embrace the untapped possibilities that our later years can offer. The most current research and data reveal that we stand on the brink of an age-awakening, where every stage of life holds the promise of purpose and contribution.

In the chapters ahead, I'll show you how embracing your Second Prime with a fresh approach can profoundly enhance your life and reshape our cultural narrative around aging. While society often portrays aging as a decline in value, productivity, and attractiveness, much of this decline is assumed. How we perceive and experience aging is within our control, allowing us to shape our aging journey with a vision for the future and a framework to support our success, creating the tomorrow we desire.

This book introduces key concepts that can elevate your life now, and in the future. We'll explore essential aspects like spirituality, connection, intellectual growth, purpose, intimacy, and more. We'll address the unique challenges of aging, uncover the benefits of growing older, and encourage a sense of pride in the wisdom we have collected over the years.

Here's the truth: This phase of life will be challenging, and you play a crucial role in changing the status quo around aging. Improving our collective mindset and approach can create a more fulfilling experience as we age. Like most things in life, attitude is everything. Let's focus on taking care of ourselves at every level while welcoming the decades ahead as opportunities for continued growth.

Finding your purpose may sound exhausting and cause you to feel even more overwhelmed than you already are. This is normal and expected; midlife is complex and busy. As you read further, you'll learn that your inconvenient dream is an internal north star that will powerfully center and ground you. Identifying your purpose allows you to do more, be more, and enjoy more in life. The distillation of what matters most, your gifts to the world and your purpose, will give you more of everything that life offers.

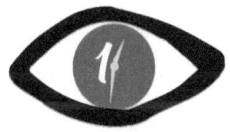

Time Crimes: A Not-So-Pretty History of Our Aging Attitudes

Time has become our most wanted fugitive. We chase it, fight it, try to capture it in bottles of serums and creams, as if aging were a crime against humanity rather than humanity's greatest triumph. Our ancestors, who rarely lived past their fourth decade, would be baffled by our modern persecution of time—this relentless pursuit of youth in an era when we've finally achieved the long-sought prize of longevity. The irony doesn't escape us; we've mastered the art of living longer while somehow forgetting how to embrace the journey. Aging is not merely a biological process—it's a mirror reflecting our deepest cultural values. While the physical reality of growing older is universal, the status of being young or old is a social construct, one that has shifted dramatically through the corridors of time.

Before the twentieth century, elders were often revered and respected for their wisdom, experience, and contributions to the community. Older adults held important roles as leaders, advisors, and mentors in many cultures. Elders were valued for their knowledge and expertise. However, rapid social and economic changes, including urbanization, industrialization, and the rise of consumer culture, contributed to a shift in attitudes toward aging. Youth and beauty became increasingly prized, while older adults were marginalized or excluded from specific social and economic opportunities.

It's difficult to pinpoint when being older was considered a negative attribute for employment. In the 1960s, it was apparent that legislation needed to protect more experienced employees. One significant development in the fight against ageism in employment was the passage of the Age Discrimination in Employment Act (ADEA) in the United States in 1967. This law prohibits employment discrimination against individuals forty years or older. It has been instrumental in providing legal protections for older workers. Several social, economic, and political factors influenced the ADEA law, highlighting the need for legal protection against age discrimination in the workplace.

The post–World War II baby boom, which created a large and influential cohort of young adults who came to define cultural norms and expectations on the social power of age, started taking shape in the latter half of the century. The rise of mass media and consumer culture further reinforced the idea that youth and beauty were essential for social and economic success. Popular media often portrays older adults in negative or stereotypical ways that powerfully influence how we respond to growing older. As our current social construct on aging continuously evolves, the relationship between age and the power it yields is in flux. Do we genuinely want to be young forever? Or do we desire to gain wisdom and cultivate the love of self and humanity while positively impacting our world?

Thirty thousand years ago, the average lifespan of our ancestors was in the late twenties or early thirties, and it remained below the age of fifty for thousands of years. In the 1800s, thanks to improved healthcare, sanitation, immunizations, and access to clean water, life expectancy doubled within ten generations. This is an exceptionally rapid increase in longevity. Although our life expectancy trajectory may slow, it's predicted that a girl born in 2011 has a one in three chance of living to the age of one hundred years old, and a boy has a one in four chance to live to one hundred years old.

Our surprisingly juxtaposed attitude is that there is a focus on how long we will live but not our quality of life. *Longevity* is a word that is thrown around in research, the wellness industry, and popular media, but without quality of life, do we really, genuinely want to live longer? Creating healthier lives needs to be an active and purposeful process; we will not parachute into health and happiness without intentionality. Attitudinal adjustments about what it means to grow into an elder require us as individuals and as a collective society to make decisions about how we want our lives to play out. We need an attitude adjustment. The good news is that positive attitudes about aging can boost longevity *and* quality of life.

A groundbreaking study published in the *Journal of Personality and Social Psychology* found that older adults with more positive attitudes about aging lived an average of 7.5 years longer than those with more negative attitudes. Let this finding sink in; attitude and outlook influence your health significantly. To give perspective, the 7.5 years of life expectancy gain is more than any other modifiable gain in health and wellness, such as quitting smoking, exercising, or improving your diet. The mind-body connection to longevity is a powerful tool to create the future you want. Our perspective on aging needs the same transformational force that science gave to longevity. However, simple truths are often hard to put into meaningful actions. It's so simple—but a negative attitude about aging is, in fact, aging.

Our relationship with aging has grown more nuanced as our lifespans have stretched beyond our ancestors' wildest dreams. While Cleopatra bathed in donkey milk and Mary, Queen of Scots preferred wine baths, their quest for eternal youth echoes through time into our modern obsession with anti-aging. We've moved from ancient beauty rituals to a full-scale assault on aging, armed with an arsenal of technologies and treatments that would make those queens marvel—yet somehow, we remain convicted by the same fears that haunted them. The real mystery isn't why we age—it's why we've criminalized a process that represents one of humanity's greatest achievements. Living longer shouldn't feel like a punishment, yet we often treat our aging bodies as if they've betrayed us. There's wisdom in caring for ourselves, in moving with intention through the decades. But there's a profound difference between nurturing our well-being and waging an endless war against time.

Each culture has anti-aging practices, reflecting a universal desire to stay young, healthy, and desirable. However, attitudes toward aging vary widely depending on cultural and individual experiences. Unfortunately, many people—especially in Western societies where youth and beauty are highly prized—harbor negative beliefs about aging. It's not just about vanity. A 2018 Pew Research Center survey revealed that nearly two-thirds of Americans are concerned about the physical changes of aging, and over half worry about cognitive decline—a fear that whispers in the shadows of our consciousness, shaping how we view our future selves.

This concern isn't entirely unfounded, yet it's often distorted by misconception. While some cognitive changes are part of normal aging—such as taking longer to learn new information or retrieve memories—research from the National Institute on Aging shows that many cognitive abilities—particularly wisdom, emotional regulation, and pattern recognition— remain stable or even improve with age. Like a living coral reef, the brain doesn't stop building—it continues creating new connections, adapting to changing environments, and developing intricate structures that become more elaborate and resilient even as decades pass. Studies have shown that older adults often excel at tasks requiring emotional intelligence and complex decision-making, drawing from their richness of life experiences.

Yet these scientific insights struggle to overcome deeply ingrained cultural narratives. A 2017 survey by the American Psychological Association found that only 29 percent of adults aged sixty and over felt positive about aging, while 55 percent were neutral, and 16 percent were outright negative. These beliefs aren't merely passive thoughts floating through our consciousness—they manifest as self-fulfilling prophecies, seeping into our cells and psyche.

Research published in *The Journals of Gerontology* demonstrates that negative age beliefs can accelerate cognitive decline, while positive attitudes toward aging are associated with better memory performance and increased longevity. Negative perceptions entangle themselves into our daily lives, leading to heightened stress, anxiety, social isolation, and even measurable health problems. Research published in *Journal of the American Medical Association* reveals that individuals with negative perceptions about aging experience measurably higher levels of cortisol—our body's primary stress hormone. This physiological response isn't temporary; it etches itself into our cellular memory, leading to chronic inflammation, a known precursor to numerous age-related diseases.

But here's the good news: Research shows that these attitudes can change. Interventions promoting positive aging—like exercise, social engagement, and purposeful living—can reshape our aging experience. By rejecting negative stereotypes and embracing the richness of this stage of life, we can improve our well-being and enjoy more fulfillment. Thankfully, the pro-aging movement is gaining momentum.

So, can we shift the narrative around aging from fear and decline to one of opportunity and growth? I passionately believe the answer is yes. We're on the verge of a revolution. Our attitudes about aging are overdue for disruption, stuck in outdated norms that don't reflect the increased lifespan or our desire to remain engaged contributors to society.

As Second Primers, we can help lead this shift. Changing the culture around aging requires us to actively challenge the limiting beliefs that hold us back. Many of us are unaware of how pervasive negative messages about aging are—until they affect us directly. The most impactful way to understand the harm of ageism is to live it. While society may not deliberately aim to diminish older people, unconscious biases often result in exactly that. Ageist attitudes aren't always meant to be hurtful, but they're deeply ingrained, and it's up to us to break the cycle.

The Second Prime framework encourages us to ask ourselves tough questions: Are we sidelining our dreams simply because we're older? Is it too late for bold changes? Or can we see this phase of life as a continuum of opportunity?

Changing how we see ourselves and each other is key to shifting the narrative—a transformation that begins in the mirror but ripples outward into the very fabric of society. Yes, the physical changes that come with age can be hard to accept, especially in a culture that idolizes youth. But beauty norms are evolving, and there's a growing appreciation for the beauty of longevity, with plenty of room for more progress in this arena.

The journey of aging, however, evolves differently across the gender spectrum, like parallel rivers carving distinct paths through time. Research published in *The Journals of Gerontology* reveals that while both men and women experience similar rates of cellular aging, society's lens dramatically shapes how these changes are perceived and experienced. Women typically begin to notice visible signs of aging in their mid-thirties, with collagen production declining by about 1 percent per year after age twenty. For men, this process often becomes noticeable a decade later, their skin's thicker dermal layer providing a biological buffer against time's markings.

The pressure to remain youthful and attractive weighs asymmetrically on women's shoulders, a burden quantified by sobering statistics. A 2021 study found that women spend an average of $313 per month on appearance-related products and services—nearly triple what men typically invest. The cosmetic industry estimates that by age fifty, women will have spent over $150,000 on anti-aging products alone. Could you imagine if we invested that money in more than our appearance? At the same time, men's spending remains relatively constant throughout their lives.

Yet the disparities run deeper than surface-level investments. Men often experience aging as a gain in wisdom and power, their gray hair and laugh lines interpreted as marks of distinction—battle scars from life's adventures that enhance rather than diminish their perceived value. A man in his fifties or sixties may be seen as distinguished, his market value in professional spheres often peaking during these decades. Meanwhile, women of the same age frequently face what researchers term the "double standard of aging," where identical signs of maturity are interpreted as decline rather than development.

This uneven aging experience reflects both personal choices and systemic patterns throughout our social consciousness. Like a river shaped by the landscape it traverses, our experience of aging is profoundly influenced by the cultural terrain through which we navigate our later years.

For men, gray hair and laugh lines can enhance attractiveness, but for women, these same signs of aging are often viewed as something to hide or fix. This double standard underscores the need for a cultural shift. Celebrating the human form at every stage of life is a powerful way to challenge the status quo. Learning to see ourselves with kindness and compassion allows us to extend that same generosity to others. As we rewrite our relationship with time, we're not just changing personal narratives—we're creating new possibilities for every generation that follows. The verdict on aging isn't set in stone; it's up for appeal, and we're both the judges and the witnesses in this transformative case.

Taking care of ourselves isn't admitting defeat in the battle against aging—it's choosing to be an active participant in our own evolution. The goal isn't to surrender to it but to dance with it gracefully. Like learning any unfamiliar new steps, there's beauty in both the stumbles and the fluid moments. This isn't about giving up or giving in; it's about giving ourselves permission to age differently than generations before us. We can simultaneously embrace our maturity and maintain our vitality, understanding that these aren't contradictions but complementary steps in life's choreography.

The real transformation begins when we shift our investment from fighting time to befriending it. Imagine redirecting those resources—both financial and emotional—into experiences that nourish not just our appearance, but our whole being. What if instead of battling wrinkles, we cultivated laugh lines through joy? What if rather than hiding our gray hair, we focused on keeping our minds vibrant and engaged? This isn't an argument for neglect, it's an invitation to expand our definition of self-care beyond the superficial. Taking care of ourselves isn't admitting defeat in the battle against aging but rather a well rounded approach to supporting our wholeness inside and out.

Challenge: Review Your Mindset

How we choose to age, both in our words and actions, can reshape what successful aging looks like—not just for ourselves but for society. As we embark on this journey, use these questions to start examining your biases around age and aging. Noticing when certain thoughts come up and where they come from is the first step to shifting the narrative.

- Examine your social media feeds. How often do you see youth and beauty linked to a specific age? Are older individuals celebrated for their uniqueness, or are they minimized or overly filtered? When you read an article, how often is the focus on the person's physical appearance versus the contribution they make? Do you see a disparity between how women are portrayed when they are in their Second Prime?
- Pay attention to how often you use or hear negative language about aging regarding yourself and others—even in humor. When you catch yourself, pause and reframe your thoughts. Focus on the growth, wisdom, and experience that come with age. This shift can influence not just you but everyone around you.

Inconvenient Dreams: The Messengers
We Try to Ignore

Ahh, mirrors and hips, they don't lie. Their honesty can feel particularly inconvenient as the years pass, but perhaps we've been asking them the wrong questions. While they reflect the undeniable changes time brings, they can't show us the wisdom we've earned, the stories we carry, or the dreams still waiting to unfold. Aging isn't just about what we see reflected back at us—it's about what we choose to do with all we've learned along the way.

Like those truthful mirrors, our inner landscape reflects both what we've become and what we're becoming. Each line earned, each subtle shift in our physical form, carries a story of experience, of choices made and paths taken. And just as we learn to look beyond surface reflections, we must learn to listen to the deeper truths our lives are trying to tell us.

Admittedly, I have both conscious and unconscious biases about aging. This is normal. Our society has ingrained dread and shame of aging so deeply in us that it takes an intentional and consistent effort to choose an alternative mindset. But here's what decades of living have taught me: The beliefs we carry about aging are like old maps drawn for territories that no longer exist. The landscape of later life has transformed, yet our cultural narrative remains stuck in outdated assumptions. The reflexive thought that aging sucks is one we've all harbored—it's right there in this book's title. But what if the real question isn't whether aging sucks, but rather if how we've been approaching it sucks?

Yes, aging comes with physical, emotional, and societal

changes—some undeniably challenging. It's okay to acknowledge these shifts, to feel their weight and meaning. Much of today's commerce thrives on making us feel inadequate, capitalizing on every perceived flaw, and urging us to wage an impossible war against time itself. The global marketing machine would have us spend billions trying to erase the very evidence of our lived experience.

But what if we've been looking at this all wrong? What if these years—this Second Prime—aren't about loss and limitation but about possibility and purpose? We—the elders, the wise ones—are not just survivors of time's passage; we are the carriers of hard-won wisdom, the holders of stories that need telling, the dreamers whose visions have been tempered and clarified by experience. Our society needs us to show up as sources of wisdom and purpose. The shift from "aging sucks" to "I am in the age of new opportunity" isn't just semantic—it's transformative.

Of course, adopting this Second Prime mindset may feel unfamiliar and impossible, and you might even resist it at first by thinking that getting older is mostly a negative experience. True transformation is complex and demands consistent effort, especially when it requires us to challenge deeply held beliefs. Most of us carry a list of things we wish we'd improved about ourselves; if we haven't accomplished it by now, time is ticking by. We may want to throw up our hands, thinking it's just too late, it's time to sideline ourselves. The key to your Second Prime transformation is to reconnect with or discover your most sacred and authentic identity—more on this later.

To navigate your Second Prime effectively, you must first unlearn and rewire negative assumptions and intentionally redefine your mindset, goals, and behaviors. As we collectively engage in this transformative work, the public rebranding of aging will unfold naturally. The media, marketers, and commerce will adapt, mirroring the new reality we create through our actions. By embodying the vitality of our Second Prime, we can inspire society to embrace this evolved perspective on aging.

We all carry within us inconvenient dreams—the ones that refuse to be silenced despite our best efforts to ignore them. They arrive uninvited and stay, making themselves at home in our consciousness until we finally pay attention. But to understand these dreams' persistent call, we must first recognize their source: our purpose in life (PIL).

These dreams that we've labeled inconvenient are profound messengers from our deeper selves. Like persistent whispers that refuse to be silenced by the noise of daily life, they carry the seeds of our most authentic future. The very qualities that make them feel inconvenient—their persistence, their demand for attention, their refusal to fit neatly into our carefully ordered lives—are precisely what make them valuable guides for our Second Prime journey.

Purpose isn't another achievement to pursue or goal to reach. It's the current that runs beneath every meaningful moment of our lives, transforming ordinary days into expressions of something deeper. When we align with this purpose, our inconvenient dreams shift from background whispers to clear guidance, showing us the path to our truest life.

Research reveals that living with purpose doesn't just enrich our emotional world—it helps preserve our cognitive function as we age, as if our brain itself thrives when we're aligned with meaning. Your purpose, like the inconvenient dreams it generates, grows and evolves with you. As founder of the Modern Elder Academy Chip Conley observes, purpose works on two levels—the overarching vision (the big "P") that shapes our life's direction, and the daily moments (the little "p") where we bring that vision to life.

These dreams show up differently for each of us. Maybe they surface in your persistent desire to teach, even when it means reimagining your entire career. Perhaps they appear in your drive to create spaces where others feel understood, or in your dedication to nurturing your family's growth despite the personal costs. Some find their inconvenient dreams pushing them to advocate for change, while others discover them in quieter moments—in deep listening, creating beauty, or being fully present for others.

Your inconvenient dreams aren't about meeting expectations or following predetermined paths. They're about recognizing and honoring your unique contribution to the world. And yes, they're inconvenient—the truth often is. But in that very inconvenience lies their power to transform not just your life, but the lives of those around you.

New work by Patricia Boyle and colleagues at the Rush Alzheimer's Disease Center suggests that PIL could be neuroprotective (brain-preserving). A seven-year study followed more than nine hundred older people at risk for dementia and found that those with a high PIL were only half as likely to develop Alzheimer's disease than those with a low PIL. The data held up even after controlling for demographics, depressive symptoms, personality vulnerabilities, social network size, and several chronic medical conditions. Those studied were also 30 percent less likely to develop mild cognitive impairment, a condition characterized by minor cognitive deficits that could (but doesn't always) progress to Alzheimer's.

Living with purpose doesn't mean the clouds will part and your life will always be sunny. But it offers something far more valuable: an internal compass that remains steady even when the path ahead seems unclear. When difficulties arise, you'll be guided by something larger, a protective shield that comes from inside, providing intrinsic resilience and emotional gratification.

Interestingly, the more passion you have for an activity, the more your daily life is infused with physiological and physical vitality. Linking your identity to your PIL is an essential connection to this internal wellspring. It's where your genius lives. When you find the thing that inspires you, the mental and physical energy needed to do the work will arrive, I assure you, no matter how busy or tired you are.

Your Second Prime arrives with a particular gift: the clarity to finally hear what your life has been trying to tell you all along. Those dreams you've labeled inconvenient—the ones that refuse to fade despite decades of practical choices—are now knocking with renewed urgency.

The timing is no coincidence. In your First Prime, life's immediate demands—career building, family raising, identity establishing—often drowned out these deeper callings. But now, standing on the foundation of accumulated wisdom, you're uniquely positioned to understand what these persistent dreams have been trying to tell you.

What makes this moment especially powerful is the growing body of research supporting what many have intuitively known: pursuing these authentic callings isn't just emotionally fulfilling—it's biologically beneficial. A groundbreaking University of Michigan study of over six thousand adults revealed that living with strong purpose significantly reduces mortality rates. When you align with your inconvenient dream, your body responds on a cellular level: inflammation decreases, sleep deepens—it's as if every fiber of your being recognizes this return to authenticity.

There's a delightful linguistic coincidence here: "Inconvenient dreams" can be abbreviated as ID, the same shorthand psychologists use for the primal, instinctual part of your psyche (the id) and your photo ID, your identity. Isn't that fitting? These ID dreams form the very core of your identity—they're what you stand for when no one's watching, the raw material of your authentic self, as unique and unrepeatable as a fingerprint. Far from mere nocturnal distractions, these dreams are your deepest identity signing its name. Like DNA itself, they contain the essential code of who you are and what you're here to contribute. They emerge not from external expectations or societal pressures but from your innermost self. Whether it's creating a community program that transforms lives, sharing wisdom through educating, or bringing beauty to forgotten spaces—the scale doesn't matter. What matters is that it's genuinely yours, an authentic expression of your deepest values in action.

This is what makes your Second Prime so extraordinary. It's not just another chapter but potentially the most meaningful one. You now have the perspective to recognize what's enormously important, the wisdom to appreciate the gift of time, and the courage to finally embrace those dreams you once deemed too inconvenient to pursue.

In our earlier years, chasing external approval, status, success, or the illusion of it, was all consuming. But this new phase of life is a chance to let go of those hollow pursuits. The inconvenient dream asks you to be brutally honest with yourself. What are you pretending not to know? Are your daily actions aligned with what truly makes your soul come alive?

The beauty of this dream is that it doesn't have to be about saving the world. But it *must* be about authenticity—something that genuinely matters to you. And the wonderful thing about aging is that it forces us to stop lying to ourselves. It's liberating. The older we get, the less we can fake it, and that's a true gift.

Pursuing your inconvenient dream doesn't just enhance your emotional well-being; it affects you physiologically. When you align with your purpose, your body responds. Stress levels drop, inflammation reduces, and your overall cellular health improves. It's like the universe starts working in tandem with your efforts, bringing opportunities and opening doors you couldn't have imagined. The feel-good hormone and neurotransmitter dopamine is increased when you are engaging with your purpose. This hormone is associated with motivation, pleasure, and reward, and it plays a vital role in memory and learning.

When you pursue a meaningful dream, your brain releases more of this high-vibe chemical, giving you the energy and motivation to keep going. Living with purpose and following your inconvenient dream isn't just about feeling good—it's about thriving in your Second Prime. It's a path to greater fulfillment, deeper meaning, and better health. When you embrace your inconvenient dream, you're changing your own life and contributing to the world in ways that can ripple out far beyond your immediate reach.

So, ask yourself: *What have I been putting off in my First Prime, deeming it too inconvenient, too much, or too impractical?* This is the time to dust it off, look at it with fresh eyes, and give it the attention it deserves. You might just find that this inconvenient dream is the key to unlocking the next, most vibrant time of your life.

Start small. Take one step toward your dream, however minor it may seem. Make time for contemplation and self-discovery. Persistence and dedication are the keys to success, and by breaking through self-limiting beliefs, you'll find your way to your true, authentic self.

Pursuing your inconvenient dream is not about achieving perfection or immediate success. It's about the journey toward growth and self-discovery. Embrace failures as lessons, celebrate small victories, and keep moving toward your vision.

Challenge: Uncovering Your Inconvenient Dream

Your inconvenient dream matters because it represents what you genuinely want to contribute during this vital stage of life. Starting small is fine. What matters is taking that first step toward what calls to you most strongly. Find a quiet moment to sit with these questions. Whether you reflect silently or write your thoughts in a journal (which often reveals insights that mere thinking doesn't uncover), honor your own process. Take your time. This isn't a test or task to complete. It's an exploration of what matters most to you now, in this season of life.

- **Heart's Truth:** What persistent idea or desire keeps returning, even when you try to dismiss it? What would bring you deep fulfillment, regardless of how impractical it might seem?

- **Past Dreams:** Which dreams have you set aside, convincing yourself the moment has passed? Consider them again, this time with the wisdom and perspective you've gained.

- **The Waiting Dream:** What have you postponed for years to make room for other priorities? What would it mean to give it space in your life now?

- **Undefined Urgency:** Do you feel a strong pull toward something you can't quite name? Pay attention to this restlessness. It often points toward meaningful change.

- **Personal Growth:** Which dreams would challenge you to expand beyond your current capabilities? The ones that make you slightly uncomfortable often hold the most potential.

- **Honest Doubts:** What specific fears or uncertainties hold you back? Write them down clearly. Understanding your resistance is the first step to moving past it.

- **Daily Reality:** How might you begin pursuing your dream alongside your current responsibilities? Small, consistent actions create lasting change.

- **New Territory:** What skills or knowledge would you need to develop? Consider this learning process part of the journey.

- **True Expression:** Which dreams align most closely with your core values? Look for the ones that feel authentic, not just impressive.

- **Ripple Effect:** How could pursuing your dream create positive change beyond your own life? Sometimes our most personal choices have unexpected ways of influencing and inspiring others.

- **Support System:** Who encourages your growth and believes in your potential? Spend time with those who support your vision, while maintaining healthy boundaries with those who don't.

Beyond the Map: When Purpose Becomes Your North Star

There's a moment that arrives, often in the quiet of an ordinary day, when we first notice the shifting ground beneath our feet. The carefully constructed timeline of our First Prime—with its predictable markers of success and achievement—begins to feel like a map to a territory we've already explored. Then, somewhere between crossing off the hundredth to-do list item and scheduling yet another dentist appointment, it hits us: We've been diligently following life's prescribed path, only to discover that reaching all the right destinations hasn't led us where we truly want to go.

Remember how predictable it all seemed? School, career, relationships, maybe kids, definitely taxes—each milestone was a silent promise that we were doing life right. But here's what no one tells you about following all the rules: You wake up one morning and realize you've been so busy checking boxes that you've forgotten to check in with yourself.

It's that head-snapping moment of clarity when we realize this is all there is . . . unless we decide it isn't. This is when we first glimpse what's possible in our Second Prime: not a predetermined set of expectations, but an invitation to finally shape our lives around what truly matters. The question isn't whether we've followed the right path; it's whether we're ready to create our own.

This is when the need for a deep, intrinsic purpose in life (PIL) emerges with unmistakable clarity. The checklist mentality that carried us through our First Prime, the one that promised fulfillment through achievement, begins to ring hollow. We find ourselves craving something more substantial than the next accomplishment, something that connects us to our deeper selves rather than just adding another line to our resume.

In our First Prime, the gates we pass through have a reassuring predictability. These stages carry a sense of momentum, each promising something fulfilling up ahead. High school flows into college or work, relationships take shape, careers progress, and, in many cases, families form. This rhythm feels almost comforting, carrying us forward with a structure that provides meaning and identity. Time feels vast, and the future appears endlessly open. Many of us rush to the next stage, eagerly anticipating life's milestones like collectibles on a journey, buoyed by the excitement of what's new and untested. Early adulthood feels almost outside time's grip; there's always more to be done and endless tomorrows to lean on.

The need for profound and deep connections with ourselves and others offers us an opportunity to break free from the checklist life and embark on a more intentional, purpose-driven journey. We no longer settle for enough; we are ready to step into a life that resonates deeply with our values and aspirations. By stepping off the societal path, we can discover the freedom to carve our unique journey, fostering growth, joy, and a purpose that is truly our own.

As we enter our Second Prime, it's crucial to recognize how our past, with all its twists and turns, impacts this new phase. Our early years often follow a well-worn path, but what if we floundered or felt adrift back then? If you've ever felt you underachieved, left potential untapped, or simply missed out, you're not alone. I often reflect on how much more I could have accomplished in my First Prime. This feeling can leave a lingering sense of shame, but it's not a dead end; instead, it fuels the drive to embrace our Second Prime with renewed purpose. The experiences and insights we've gained are valuable tools to finally pursue our inconvenient dreams.

As time progresses, something subtle yet profound begins to shift. Goals and priorities that once seemed vital begin to fade, often replaced by a gnawing question: *Now what?* In our formative years, our purpose was simply growing up, establishing ourselves, and achieving milestones. But those ego and acquisition-driven pursuits lose their allure as we grow and acquire wisdom. We find ourselves looking for a deeper sense of meaning and fulfillment, a purpose that speaks directly to who we are today. Life coach Barbara Waxman calls this transitional stage *middlescence*, a period in our forties to sixties marked by a powerful desire to redefine purpose. And just as our sense of purpose shifts, so does our relationship with time itself.

We reach a point where many of life's firsts have passed, and the days become more routine and predictable. This can make time feel finite, almost urgent, as if possibilities are dwindling. When we see time as limited, our sense of potential shrinks instead of expanding. Society often reinforces this, allowing us to believe it's too late to change and that aging means we've missed our chance for impact. But this is simply a mindset trap. What if, instead, we saw this time as one of freedom, where the question becomes: *If not now, when?*

Here's a fascinating insight about time: It can feel like it's dragging on or racing by depending on the neurochemicals at play, especially dopamine. Dopamine is the brain's reward-system driver, influencing our perception of time, drive, and happiness. This is crucial because, when harnessed, it can infuse our days with meaning and fulfillment. However, it's also tied to behaviors that distract or detract from a life of purpose. Dopamine gives us a sense of reward, yes, but it doesn't distinguish between rewards that serve us and those that don't. It's why instant gratification can pull us in, whether through screens, food, shopping, or other quick-fix distractions. This isn't just a concern for the young; as we age, especially if we're dissatisfied with our lives, these dopamine hits can lure us away from what truly matters.

The real power of dopamine lies in directing it toward activities that add depth and joy. Experiencing something new, even in small ways, can bring a surge of excitement that makes time feel expansive. These micro-adventures, whether they're learning a skill, exploring a new place, or even having a meaningful conversation, spark natural euphoria. So, how do we create meaningful moments that feel purposeful? By aligning our actions with values that uplift us and investing in people and activities that bring out our best.

Recognizing our relationship with time lets us make conscious decisions instead of allowing the routine lull us into losing hours and days on things that don't fit our vision of the future. When we understand the role of dopamine, we can start fostering pro-dopamine habits, like spending time with people who inspire us, engaging in pursuits that offer accomplishment and meaning, and bringing fresh experiences into our lives. These choices help build a future that aligns with our deeper purpose, transforming the Second Prime into a period of growth, fulfillment, and joy.

Unlike the demands of youth, your Second Prime is not driven by ego or status. Instead, it's motivated by purpose and a desire to contribute to something greater than yourself. Earlier in life, many of us follow a road map—college, career, marriage, family, mortgages—that sweeps us into midlife, often leaving us feeling exhausted and unfulfilled. Despite achievements, we may wonder: *Is this all there is?* This is the quiet but real discontent of midlife.

The Happiness Curve

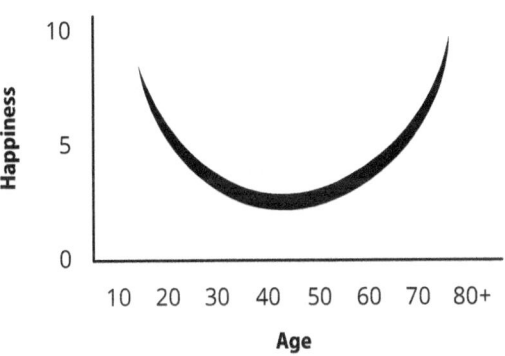

By the time you reach midlife, your tolerance for nonsense plummets. Buh-bye BS! Yet, oddly, it's not impatience but a sharpened clarity about what truly matters. As my friend Abby says, "The ability to tolerate BS nosedives in your forties, and by fifty, you're in a no-BS zone." This shift is more than liberating; it's transformative, stripping away unnecessary obligations and inviting you to engage only with what aligns with your core values.

This clarity arrives like dawn breaking over familiar terrain, revealing contours you never noticed in the dim light of your First Prime. It's not that you've become less tolerant. You've become more attuned to the quiet voice of authenticity that's been whispering all along. Each *no* to what doesn't serve you becomes a *yes* to what deeply matters. Each boundary you draw creates space for something more meaningful to flourish. Think of it as finally removing a pair of glasses you didn't know you were wearing— lenses created from others' expectations, societal pressures, and inherited beliefs about what makes a life worthwhile. The world may appear less accommodating at first, but it becomes infinitely more real. Your time, your energy, your presence—these are no longer resources to be parceled out to the highest bidder of habit, obligation, or expectation. They become sacred elements of a life chosen with intention.

Imagine standing at the bottom of a valley, looking up. This is where many of us find ourselves in our forties and early fifties, and it's the lowest point of what researchers call the U-shaped happiness curve. But here's what makes this valley unique: It's not a place of permanent residence but a launching pad. This dip in life satisfaction isn't a cruel joke of middle age; it's often the very catalyst that propels us toward our most authentic life.

The valley holds a secret: It's where we finally shed the weight of others' expectations. It's where we stop trying to climb the mountain someone else chose for us and begin to chart our own course. Those who emerge from this valley with renewed joy aren't just survivors of a midlife "crisis." They're architects of their Second Prime, using their hard-won wisdom to build lives of deeper purpose and connection.

Why does this happen? For one, there's a distinct confidence in knowing yourself better and accepting yourself more than ever. We have faced life's ups and downs, tried on countless roles, and learned through trial and error what fits and what doesn't. By this age, standing up for yourself or contradicting others is less about confrontation and more about honoring your truth. It feels so good to be authentic, like a really cozy, comfortable sweater. After all, years of experience help you filter out distractions and maintain focus on what is profoundly important.

For example, consider social situations that once might have felt obligatory. In your twenties or thirties, you may have been compelled to attend every social gathering or say yes to every request for fear of missing out or disappointing someone. By your Second Prime, however, these social obligations transform: You value quality over quantity, choosing experiences that nurture your well-being rather than drain it. The power to say no is strengthened by the knowledge that your time is limited and priceless.

This no-BS approach doesn't mean cynicism or hostility. On the contrary, it's a positive reinforcement of your self-love. The emotional freedom that comes with age means you can love others more fully without getting tangled in their expectations.

This freedom is directly linked to time's increasingly precious nature. With fewer years ahead than behind, you start measuring opportunities and choices by their potential for meaning and joy, not by societal standards or surface-level gains. The ticking clock can heighten anxiety for some, as physical changes and life's finite nature become undeniable. But it also builds the urgency to spend your days meaningfully, a call to live purposefully rather than merely coast.

Social posturing, keeping up appearances, or striving for achievements that are not in congruence with your purpose lose their luster. With wisdom as a compounding asset, you care more about aligning with your values than impressing others. The fear of what others think diminishes, replaced by a sense of satisfaction in the person you've become—a version of yourself that is finally, fully you.

Remember, in your Second Prime, you are wiser, more innovative, emotionally intelligent, and equipped with more experience than ever. One quality that sustains this growth is curiosity. While experience is an asset, curiosity keeps you from slipping into complacency. Embracing curiosity as you age helps counter the pitfalls of routine and opens your mind to innovative ideas, perspectives, and possibilities. Curiosity about the world, new experiences, and yourself keeps you flexible and open to growth. You're following leads, asking questions, and diving into what fascinates you without fear of looking foolish. Just think of your purpose as a truffle waiting to be discovered, unearthed, and savored; and you are the truffle pig, seeking it out with a spirit of discovery.

A growth mindset—an inquisitive mindset that embraces learning, resilience, and open-mindedness—is transformative at any age. It means meeting challenges with an open heart, learning from setbacks, celebrating others' successes, and remaining adaptable. This mindset enables you to evolve each year and decade, growing more discerning and ingenious as you move forward.

The midlife low can be reframed as an invitation to reconnect with your essence. What have you tolerated or kept up appearances for in the past that now feels unnecessary? This stage offers the chance to align your life with the things that give you energy and focus. In this process, you discover that courage and curiosity aren't relics of youth but tools for continual reinvention. They're the vehicles through which your inconvenient dreams—your deeper purpose—come into clearer focus.

While aging compresses our sense of time, it also clarifies priorities. The beauty of this stage is that we can let go of the illusions that used to consume us and intentionally choose a life rooted in what truly matters. Living purposefully demands commitment and courage, but it also invites a deep sense of satisfaction.

The journey into your Second Prime isn't just about leaving things behind. It's about conscious choosing. Each belief we release creates space for a new truth to take root. Each priority we shift allows a deeper purpose to emerge. These aren't just mental exercises; they're acts of gentle revolution, small but powerful declarations of who we're becoming. As you approach these challenges, treat them not as items on yet another to-do list but as doorways into your own wisdom.

Challenge: Thoughtfully Question Yourself

Take time with each question. Let your answers surprise you. Allow yourself to hear the truth that rises from a place deeper than thought.

- List three beliefs or priorities you no longer have from your First Prime and how that makes you feel.
  - Example: I do not need to compare myself with others to determine my worth; this realization makes me feel free and confident.
- List three new beliefs/commitments/actions you want to cultivate in your Second Prime and how you want to feel when you embody them.
  - Example: I will dedicate myself to following through on my purpose in life and keeping promises to myself. By committing to my inconvenient dream, I will align with what I stand for, which will give me a feeling of deep contentment.

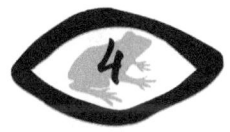

The Midlife "Crisis": And Why It Is Really an Invitation

Picture a room in London, 1957. A Canadian psychoanalyst named Elliott Jaques stands before his colleagues at the British Psychoanalytical Society, about to name something millions have felt but never quite understood. As he describes the profound restlessness that visits us in our middle years, heads begin to nod. In that moment, the midlife crisis was born—not as the commercialized cliché it would become, but as a recognition of a deeply human experience: the complex reckoning with what we've built and what still calls to us from the horizon of possibility.

Through his systematic study of 310 artists, composers, writers, and scientists, Jaques identified a distinct pattern: An individual's creative work often underwent significant transformation during their mid-thirties to early forties. He observed how these intense feelings surfaced in diverse ways. In some cases, it appeared as extreme depression, hypochondria, spiritual awakening, or even wild attempts to reclaim youth, like promiscuity. In less expressive personalities, these struggles showed up in smaller, more subtle ways. Yet, they reflected a shared experience: grappling with what one has (or hasn't) achieved and reconciling this with a dwindling sense of possibility.

The modern midlife crisis became a familiar trope and commercialized concept, especially in the Western world. As we transitioned away from physically demanding, life-shortening work, middle adulthood, or middlescence, became a luxury afforded by improved living standards. And with that luxury came complex, sometimes unexpected, challenges. No longer are most of us confined to lives spent toiling in fields or factories with an expected lifespan capped at fifty or sixty years. Instead, we're tasked with navigating a new phase of life marked by growing contradictions. In this period, we experience gains in self-awareness, emotional intelligence, and interpersonal wisdom. Yet, we can also feel profound losses: shifts in identity, physical vitality, and even relationships.

The prevalence of the crisis messaging has shaped a perspective that focuses heavily on these perceived losses. Companies have capitalized on this narrative, offering rejuvenation or youth preservation in products, diets, or activities that promise to stave off signs of aging and provide relief from the pangs of time. But the so-called crisis is only part of the story. When we look beyond the labels and clichés, we find that midlife offers tremendous growth and opportunity if we approach it intentionally. There are indeed gains alongside the losses, which can be profoundly fulfilling and affirming if we pursue them purposefully.

Let's explore the potent combination of experience, wisdom, and purpose at an age when we can choose to wield our maturity for personal growth and even more significant societal change. Yet, many of us stumble here, falling into traps of our own making. Some enter a period of recklessness, self-centeredness, or aimless grasping. This is a misguided attempt to reclaim a sense of direction, vitality, and possibility that feels like it's slipping away. We've all seen examples of this in friends or loved ones—flashy sports cars, affairs, escapism through alcohol, or excessive plastic surgery. In their search to feel relevant, powerful, or simply alive, people too often take paths that disrupt their lives without fulfilling their deeper needs.

Many people who experience a midlife crisis struggle with a loss of potential, often accompanied by the feeling that time is running out. This can feel overwhelming and unsettling, causing them to seek anything that brings them joy or a sense of power. This desire to feel vibrant and meaningful is inescapable; it's part of the human experience. But it can become destructive when we misinterpret or overreach in our attempt to re-establish those feelings.

It's important to distinguish the blurred lines between genuine self-discovery and escapist reinvention. For example, a familiar scenario is the friend who decides, in midlife, to find themselves. In one case, my friend shared a story of a woman who left her financially stable, family-oriented life, abandoning her spouse and splitting up her family. To her, this was the noble pursuit of her purpose; to others, it looked like a midlife crisis in disguise— perhaps it was both. However, purpose should not require blowing up other people's lives. Finding purpose should not be an excuse for unchecked self-indulgence or a reason to discard our responsibilities in the pursuit of self-satisfaction.

Instead, true purpose demands self-accountability. While the cultural script for this phase of life is unclear, finding purpose in our Second Prime should feel more like an act of integration than one of rebellion.

In your Second Prime, a profound opportunity emerges: the chance to align who you truly are with what the world deeply needs. This alignment—what we call PIL—becomes the bridge between crisis and transformation. When you're feeling lost, your inconvenient dream, your PIL, illuminates the path forward, offering an alternative to the familiar crisis narrative of midlife.

Let's examine how misalignment drives us toward those midlife crises and how pursuing your purpose can be the healthier, more fulfilling alternative. To truly grow, we must move beyond viewing aging as a process of decline. Embracing this new life phase requires maturity, wisdom, and a genuine commitment to find purpose beyond what's fleeting or shallow.

It's crucial to understand that PIL is not a get-out-of-crisis-free card. Sometimes, our yearning for purpose can deceive us into believing we're on a noble path when, in reality, we're avoiding responsibilities or chasing illusions. Purpose is a powerful compass, but only when used with integrity and honesty. Without a clear, realistic foundation, the "purposeful" path can end up causing as much harm as a crisis-driven reaction. To avoid these pitfalls, we must approach PIL with clear self-accountability. Ask yourself: *Is this action aligned with my values and commitments? Am I being honest about my motivation?*

Finding true purpose doesn't mean neglecting or abandoning the people and roles that are important to us. Instead, it should deepen our commitment to them in meaningful ways.

Transitioning into a purpose-driven life can be uncomfortable, but this discomfort is a vital signal of growth. Like a muscle that strengthens under strain, your inner life expands when you grapple with discomfort rather than avoid it. True purpose asks us to grow, deepen, and accept that there are unexplored facets of ourselves. In all its complexity, embracing aging can offer a meaningful, less crisis-ridden path through midlife.

Consider the idea of striving without struggling. Striving in this sense is a matter of developing alignment and coherence. When your purpose matches your values and actions, discomfort becomes manageable or even productive, a desired difficulty. The journey to find purpose may require hard choices and sacrifice. Still, it also offers profound rewards, like a deeper, more genuine satisfaction than fleeting indulgences ever could.

One of the biggest misconceptions about aging is that it automatically leads to loss, decline, and irrelevance. But a purpose-driven life has the power to reshape these perceptions entirely. When your life has meaning and direction, physical changes—like the lines on your face or the graying of your hair—are less disappointing and less threatening. You're more than your appearance or status; you're a person with value, knowledge, and an impact to make.

Midlife is a time to nurture and develop intangible qualities that don't fade with age. Courage, compassion, curiosity, resilience, and wisdom all grow stronger over time. By shifting our focus inward, we transcend the limitations of our ego and move closer to our soul, which is where true joy resides.

As you move into your Second Prime, ask yourself regularly: *What do I stand for?* The values and virtues that define you become your internal compass, guiding your choices and actions. Those who embrace their PIL discover that each challenge and change in midlife serves as a refining fire, clarifying their purpose and strengthening their character. And those who avoid their purpose often find themselves swept up in crises as their inner compass becomes muddied by regret, envy, or discontent.

The key to navigating midlife is staying connected to this compass. If viewed as a friend rather than an enemy, your discomfort signals where you need to grow. With the self-awareness that comes from purposeful living, you'll find joy not in escaping the changes that come with age but in facing them and embracing them fully.

Transition offers us a unique opportunity to develop the wisdom that comes from experience and to apply that wisdom toward something greater than ourselves. Unlike youth, which prioritizes energy and novelty, your Second Prime is about depth. As we age, the world begins to slow down, not because we're becoming less capable, but because we're becoming more discerning. Our priorities shift from endless newness to meaningful impact. There's no longer a need to chase every opportunity or prove every point; instead, we can focus on what truly matters, actions and choices that leave a lasting imprint.

If youth is wasted on the young, don't let wisdom be wasted on you. Let the Second Prime be your time to align purpose with action and use your skills to guide you toward a life of joy, connection, and fulfillment. The decisions you make now, based on values and purpose rather than fear or ego, set the stage for a life well-lived, not just longer-lived.

During our lives, we experience transitions—some subtle, some seismic. Often, these shifts unearth an unease that's easy to dismiss or bury, but as the thirteenth-century spiritual master and poet Rumi suggests, our pain is a messenger. By midlife, we possess the hard-won wisdom to pause and listen. This gift allows us to step back and assess ourselves from new angles. Midlife equips us with perspective—a capacity to look beyond immediate anxieties and see who we are with greater clarity and acceptance.

This clarity extends to our cognitive abilities in specific, measurable ways. Research shows that while processing speed may decrease, our crystallized intelligence—the ability to use knowledge, experience, and learned skills—continues to strengthen well into our sixties and seventies. Our pattern recognition and complex problem-solving abilities often peak in middle age, providing a clearer sense of our true values and goals.

And so, this midlife crisis is not a crisis at all but an awakening. It's a nudge from within, a call to realign our lives with our inner truth and purpose. You may feel the dull ache of unmet possibilities as if something has yet to be answered. Rather than seeing this as a flaw, consider it a golden opportunity—a prompt from your deeper self to ask: *What's next?* This question creates an opening, a fertile space for growth and potential that's perhaps more meaningful now than ever before. If you find that joy or satisfaction from past pursuits has faded or that your values are shifting, let that signal inspire not unsettle you. This internal opening is a rare moment of recalibration, a time when you can step back from society's outdated narrative that midlife means stepping aside by making choices that are truly yours.

In truth, the restless unease you may experience is your purpose calling out. When we're out of tune with our authentic identity, it shows up in ways we often label negative—discomfort, boredom, irritability. But these are guideposts—not stop signs— pointing you toward a life that aligns with your inner values. Your soul is asking you to look within, to uncover what makes your life feel rich with meaning. The secret to thriving in midlife is simple but profound: pursue your purpose. This is the ultimate anti-aging secret, igniting a vitality that not only impacts your energy but your entire outlook.

Marcus Aurelius captured it well: "Look within. Within is the fountain of good, and it will ever bubble up if thou wilt ever dig." This is your moment to start digging.

If you're feeling overwhelmed or stuck, it's a good sign—it means your inconvenient dream is waiting for you. Midlife allows us to answer its call with experience and wisdom that eluded us when we were young. While the fast-paced ambition of youth may have faded, we're left with something more valuable: depth and wisdom. As Chip Conley describes it, we are now *wisdom workers*, equipped with life's greatest asset to offer a world in need.

Your Second Prime offers a rare, precious invitation to come fully alive. The unease you feel isn't just discomfort—it's the stirring of dormant potential, a call to reawaken. Each moment of uncertainty carries within it the seeds of transformation. When you embrace this perspective, the very feelings that might have triggered a crisis become stepping stones toward purpose. Science confirms this potential: Studies consistently show that wisdom, decision-making, and even entrepreneurial success peak in our fifties and sixties. The evidence is clear—your Second Prime isn't just another life phase; it's potentially your most powerful stage for creating meaningful impact.

As you lean into this phase, remember to embrace the journey, and let it reveal the depths of your wisdom, resilience, and dreams. The world needs your gifts, and you deserve the fulfillment they bring when you give them away.

Challenge: Uncover and Nurture Your Inconvenient Dream

The feelings of restlessness and discomfort may point directly to your purpose. Here are some actionable steps you can take to uncover and nurture your inconvenient dream:

- **Identify Your Gifts:** Take inventory of your unique strengths, the skills you've gained, and the insights others recognize in you. This will illuminate areas where you can make a significant impact.

- **Rewrite Your Life's Script:** Pause to question the assumptions you hold about aging and midlife. If society tells you it's time to step back, challenge that notion. Midlife isn't the end of contribution—it's the perfect moment to reinvest your wisdom in ways that matter most.

- **Align with Your Core Values:** Reflect on the values that define you now. They may have changed since your younger years, and that's okay. Choose three to five core values that resonate with your current self and let them guide your next steps.

- **Take a Small Action Daily:** Pursue your purpose with incremental steps. This could be dedicating an hour a week to a passion project, volunteering, or reconnecting with people who inspire you. Purpose doesn't happen over-night—it grows through consistent, intentional action and curiosity.

- **Track Your Energy and Fulfillment:** Notice how you feel after each activity. Does it energize or drain you? Use these insights to refine your path toward a purpose that fuels you, even in challenging moments.

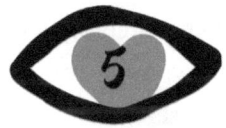

The Future You: An Inside Job

I remember the exact moment my inconvenient dream took hold—not with a thunderclap of revelation, but with a quiet, persistent question that wouldn't let go. Sitting in my favorite coffee shop, watching people rush past the window, I noticed how the older faces in the crowd seemed to carry an invisible weight, a resignation I recognized all too well and feared so deeply. The story society had written for them, for us, felt like a script I could no longer accept.

The dream that began to crystallize that morning was both terrifying and exhilarating: to fundamentally disrupt how we think about aging and ignite a movement that celebrates our midlife and beyond as periods of unprecedented potential and leadership. The voice of doubt was quick to surface: *Who are you to take this on? There are more qualified experts, more accomplished voices.*

But then I heard another voice, one that came from a deeper place. It was my future self, the woman I'm becoming, who looked back at this pivotal moment and whispered, *Why not me? Who better to contribute to this transformation than someone who refuses to accept the diminishing narrative we've been handed?*

The truth is, every movement that has ever reshaped society began with individuals who dared to question the accepted story. My future self wasn't asking me to singlehandedly revolutionize aging; she was asking me to be one of many voices, one of many lights illuminating a new path forward. She understood what I was just beginning to grasp: that our Second Prime isn't a consolation prize or a gentle fade into irrelevance but a powerful launching pad for leadership, wisdom, and profound impact.

For generations, many have embraced the narrative that age brings irrelevance, pushing wisdom and experience to the sidelines. Aging isn't the issue; it's how we approach it. We are responsible for shattering the "aging sucks" mindset by living as vibrant examples of how fulfilling our Second Prime can be. To create this transformation, we need a mindful and comprehensive approach to enhancing our later years.

Transforming your *why*—your true purpose in life—into action becomes a potent elixir for the body, mind, and soul. By committing to your inconvenient dream, you unlock a transformative potential that can revitalize every aspect of your existence. It's akin to tapping into a hidden reservoir of health, inspiration, vitality, and drive that resides within you. Slaying the dragons of your Second Prime invigorates your spirit, making you feel more alive and robust than ever before.

How you choose to age hinges on your decisions and the identity you craft during your Second Prime. One powerful question can set the course for this journey: *Will my future self thank me?* This deceptively simple question is a master key—the caliber of inquiries we pose to ourselves determines which doors of possibility swing open and which remain forever locked. By embracing positive, vitality-centric behaviors now, you set in motion a cascade of benefits that will culminate in a more joyful, life-affirming self as you approach your sixties and seventies.

This intentional cultivation of positive habits equips you with the tools to become the person you aspire to be, embodying the values that resonate most deeply with you in your Second Prime.

As we've explored, the First Prime is often a more straightforward path that leads us through the pursuit of legitimacy and adulthood, where we can drift along the currents of societal expectations. However, this passive approach falls short in your Second

Prime, where the stakes are higher and your future is on the line. In this phase, you must actively foster a mindset filled with optimism and expansive possibilities.

Create a roadmap for the life you desire that reflects your aspirations. By building an intentional plan and shifting your perspective, you will discover greater contentment and joy in the process of taking action, irrespective of the outcomes. The energy and effort you invest in your new pursuits will manifest the life you have always envisioned.

Future self-reflection is a transformative tool that can inspire change, banish procrastination, and guide us to live intentionally today for the benefit of tomorrow. Before I committed fully to my purpose—my inconvenient dream—my answer to the question, *Will my future self thank me?* was often a hesitant, *I hope so.* However, hope alone isn't a strategy; it's part of a larger, intentional plan. To truly thrive in our Second Prime, we must act purposefully, guided by a sharp vision of the life we want.

When we envision our future selves, we might picture role models like Chrissie Hynde, still performing in her seventies; Christine Lagarde, leading the European Central Bank in her sixties; or Shonda Rhimes, breaking stereotypes while transforming culture through entertainment. What sets these individuals apart isn't just their passion but their planning—a purposeful strategy for living a meaningful and engaged life.

This brings us to the importance of having a purpose in life (PIL) and a plan in life (PIL). While our purpose in life represents our *why,* our plan in life serves as the *how*—the roadmap that transforms intentions into actions and hopes into reality. Without a plan in life, our purpose can remain a distant dream.

Creating a plan in life doesn't have to be overwhelming; it's meant to be fun and joyful. It can begin with small, achievable goals and evolve from there. The key is to be intentional and strategic in our actions, aligning them with our purpose and values. This provides direction and helps maintain motivation and focus on what truly matters to us.

A thoughtfully crafted plan in life allows for flexibility and self-compassion. As you work toward your inconvenient dream, your priorities and goals may shift, offering new insights and evolving perspectives. Having a road map keeps you accountable to yourself, enabling you to adjust your course without losing sight of your overall purpose.

Planning is more than jotting down thoughts; it's an act of personal belief and a powerful tool for manifesting your future. When you commit to a plan, you create a version of yourself in sync with your dreams. This process becomes a conversation between your present self and your future self—a commitment to nurture and actively create the life you desire.

Also, the act of planning itself brings rewards. Neuroscience shows that planning stimulates the prefrontal cortex, the brain area responsible for decision-making and purposeful actions. By organizing your path, you strengthen the mental muscles that guide discipline, motivation, and resilience.

The beauty of habit formation lies in its gentle persistence. As James Clear brilliantly illustrates in *Atomic Habits*, we don't transform our lives through dramatic upheavals but through the quiet accumulation of tiny, consistent changes. Think of it like compound interest for your personal growth: Each small habit builds upon itself, creating a magnificent snowball effect that carries you toward your dreams.

I've discovered this truth in my own journey through *habit stacking*—a concept Clear suggests where you pair a new behavior with an existing habit, creating a natural trigger that bypasses willpower—that has become my daily companion.

For instance, every morning after I pour my coffee (current

habit), I spend just five minutes journaling about my future self (new habit). This simple pairing has become a sacred ritual, a daily conversation with the person I'm becoming. It's these small, intentional bridges between who we are and who we want to be that make all the difference.

There's a hidden joy in achieving small wins. Taking small steps toward a larger vision releases dopamine in a positive and healthful way; as you already know, the feel-good neurotransmitter rewards progress. It's why crossing things off a to-do list brings such satisfaction. This chemical release encourages further action and reinforces a sense of purpose that sustains us.

Planning with purpose not only fosters a sense of accomplishment but also physically benefits your brain. Studies show that those who engage in goal setting and future-oriented activities report higher satisfaction and lower stress levels. When we have a clear plan, we feel more grounded and capable of handling life's challenges. The magic often happens in focused bursts. I've fallen in love with the Pomodoro Technique—a time-management method where I give myself twenty-five-minute chunks of beautifully undistracted time where I chase my inconvenient dream with complete presence. It's amazing how these temporal boundaries actually expand our creative capacity. During these focused sessions, I often find myself entering what scientists call a *flow state*, where time seems to dissolve and possibility flourishes.

Imagine your future self, living the life you're actively planning today. Your health is strong, your relationships are rich, your mind is engaged, and your spirit is fulfilled. You're crafting this vision with each small action and thoughtful decision. Your purpose in life illuminates the way, while your plan in life creates your path.

As you take tangible steps toward realizing your inconvenient dream, your mindset about aging will shift dramatically. You will begin to see yourself through a lens of compassion, and the out-dated narrative society has imposed on aging will start to feel like a relic of the past—an ineffective marketing strategy that no longer resonates. We won't buy into it anymore!

And the science of neuroplasticity offers us an extraordinary gift: the knowledge that our brains remain malleable throughout our lives. Research from Stanford University shows that simply believing in our capacity to change actually enhances our ability to do so. When we envision our future selves and take consistent action toward becoming them, we're not just daydreaming; we're literally rewiring our neural pathways.

My future self needs me to be an engaging storyteller. So at fifty-three, I decided to get more comfortable with public speaking—not just basic presentations, but the kind of storytelling that moves audiences to action. Understanding that each practice session was literally rewiring my brain transformed my relationship with discomfort. Those butterflies in my stomach—was I feeling fear, excitement, a little of both? I no longer viewed them as warnings to retreat but signals of my brain expanding its capabilities. Every small step forward in pursuing our inconvenient dreams triggers a natural biochemical reward system.

This knowledge revolutionized how I approach challenges. When I feel that initial resistance to learning something new, whether it's mastering social media to spread my message or tackling complex research about aging, I remind myself that my brain is still eager to grow, still creating new neural pathways. Research reveals that having a powerful sense of purpose (like my mission to transform society's view of aging) actively supports brain health. When we engage in meaningful pursuits that benefit others, our brains light up with activity in regions associated with reward, learning, and emotional well-being.

Every time we choose growth over comfort, we're changing

our circumstances and physically reshaping our brains to support continued growth and adaptation. This isn't just about maintaining cognitive function. It's about thriving, about creating new possibilities well into our later years. Your future self's capacity for growth and impact may be far greater than you imagine.

This is where the rubber meets the road in our Second Prime. Every time you choose the stairs over the elevator, pick up that book instead of your phone, or have that challenging conversation you've been avoiding, you're casting a vote for your future self. These micro-moments of choice become the building blocks of your tomorrow.

Think of it like this: Each positive habit you cultivate today is writing a love letter to your future self. That morning meditation practice is telling your future self, *I want to have peace and inner strength.* That weekly dance class is saying, *I want to move with joy and less pain.* That hour spent learning a new skill is declaring, *I believe in my capacity to grow.*

When you ask, *Will my future self thank me?* let the answer be a bold proud *Yes!* You're intentionally creating a life filled with purpose, meaning, and joy in your Second Prime.

Challenge: Your Future Self's Road Map

Your future self is not some distant stranger. It's you, shaped by the thousands of tiny decisions you make today. When you feel resistance to change (and you will), pause and ask yourself: *What story do I want my future self to tell myself about this moment; what virtue will I employ to overcome resistance?*

Here's your step-by-step guide to build a life your future self will thank you for:

1. **Define Your Future Self:** Picture yourself in your Second Prime and beyond. Who are you? What are your values? What contributions have you made? What relationships do you cherish? Use these reflections to inspire an unclouded vision.

2. **Set Purpose-Driven Goals:** Define clear, achievable goals that align with your purpose. If your purpose centers on connection, your goals might include fostering deep relationships or volunteering in your community.

3. **Create Habit Bridges Through Stacking:** Master the art of habit stacking, a game-changing approach developed by James Clear. Instead of relying on willpower alone, anchor new habits to existing ones: *Before I have my morning chia pudding, I do yoga and walk the dog.* Or, *After I brush my teeth, I will do five minutes of stretching.* These natural pairings create a flow that makes transformation almost effortless. Build your stack gradually—one small victory at a time.

4. **Harness Creative Flow with Pomodoro:** Embrace the Pomodoro Technique as your creativity companion. Set your timer for twenty-five minutes of focused work, followed by a five-minute break. This rhythm honors your brain's natural capacity for deep work while preventing burnout. I've found that three or four focused Pomodoros can yield more progress than hours of scattered effort. During your breaks, move your body, hydrate, or simply breathe. These moments of pause are where inspiration often strikes.

5. **Document Your Journey:** Keep a Future Self Journal where you regularly dialogue with your older, wiser self. What would they want you to know? What choices would

they be grateful for? Let this ongoing conversation guide your daily decisions.

6. **Prioritize Small, Consistent Steps:** Planning involves daily actions, not grand gestures. Repeatedly ask yourself: *Will this decision bring me closer to the person I want to become?* Small, intentional choices lead to remarkable results.

7. **Establish a Support Network:** Surround yourself with people who share your vision or inspire you to stay on track. A dedicated support system offers encouragement and accountability.

8. **Anticipate Challenges and Build Resilience:** Aging may present difficulties, but facing challenges becomes easier with mental preparation. Cultivate resilience through self-compassion and humor.

9. **Celebrate Progress Along the Way:** Acknowledge each step you take toward your envisioned future. Celebrating milestones keeps you motivated and reminds you that every effort is part of a larger journey.

10. **Prioritize Lifelong Learning:** Engage in activities that keep your mind active and curious, whether through reading, taking courses, or learning new skills. Lifelong learning keeps you mentally sharp and adaptable.

The Biology of Authenticity: Your Cells Know When You're Lying to Yourself

Have you ever noticed how your body whispers its truth long before your mind catches up? Perhaps it's the subtle tightness in your shoulders when you're living out of alignment with your values or that inexplicable energy surge when you're pursuing something that truly matters to you. These aren't just random physical sensations—they're the profound language of your body speaking its wisdom.

Our thoughts have a powerful influence over our bodies, and our attitudes shape our experiences. Do you think your best years are behind you? Then guess what—you're right. With that belief in place, you will likely feel it's all downhill from here. Harnessing the mind-body axis is the key to accessing the power of thought, belief, and mindset to improve your aging experience. Let's say you hyper-focus on what ails you—aches, pains, chronic headaches, and so on. In this scenario, your ailments will play a starring role in your daily life. They'll impact every experience you have with the world.

Let's explore the incredible interaction between our thoughts, emotions, and physical health. This relationship profoundly affects how we age and thrive. The mind-body axis is a remarkable, interconnected network that includes systems like the nervous system, microbiome, endocrine (hormonal) system, and digestive system. Each of these plays a unique yet interdependent role in shaping our well-being. By understanding and engaging with these systems, you unlock powerful tools to enhance your quality of life in your

Second Prime, aligning body and mind to support a healthier, more fulfilling future.

The nervous system is your body's command hub, responsible for everything from conscious thought to automatic functions like breathing and heart rate. It's divided into the central nervous system (brain and spinal cord) and the peripheral nervous system, which branches out to nerves all over your body. This extensive network allows your brain to communicate with every cell, influencing how you think, feel, and respond to the world.

Within this system lies the limbic system—the emotional center of the brain, including structures like the amygdala and hippocampus, which manage deep emotions, like fear and pleasure, and survival instincts. Ever feel a surge of energy wash over you before a big event? That's your limbic system translating emotional anticipation into a physical response. Over time, patterns like chronic worry can prime the limbic system to overreact, contributing to heightened stress responses or even chronic inflammation.

When you're stressed, your brain's hypothalamus kicks off a chain reaction, sending signals through your autonomic nervous system to trigger a fight-or-flight response. Adrenaline surges, your heart rate spikes, and your body gets ready to act. This sympathetic response is strong for brief moments but, if constantly activated, can lead to health issues like high blood pressure, digestive problems, and poor sleep. Fortunately, you can help your nervous system recalibrate by incorporating practices like yoga, deep breathing, or progressive muscle relaxation. These techniques activate the parasympathetic nervous system, your body's natural rest-and-digest mode, which lowers stress and brings you back into balance. By fostering positive emotional experiences—through laughter, connection, or gratitude—you can also reshape your limbic responses, boosting resilience and well-being.

The microbiome, located primarily in your gut, is composed of trillions of bacteria and other microorganisms. It is like an internal ecosystem that influences everything from digestion to immune function and mood. Some call it the second brain because of its close communication with the brain through the gut-brain axis.

This connection is why you might feel your gut flip when you're anxious or experience stomach upset after a stressful day. The microbiome produces mood-regulating neurotransmitters like serotonin and dopamine, impacting mental and emotional health. If this delicate ecosystem is thrown off—say, by poor diet or prolonged stress—it can contribute to anxiety, depression, and digestive discomfort. Eating a diet rich in fiber, probiotics (like yogurt or sauerkraut), and prebiotics (found in foods like garlic and bananas) nourishes your microbiome, helping to stabilize your mood, clear mental fog, and strengthen your immune response. We will dive deeper into the importance of your microbiome in a forthcoming chapter.

The endocrine system, made up of glands that release hormones into the bloodstream, regulates everything from growth and metabolism to mood and sleep. Hormones like cortisol (the stress hormone), insulin (which manages blood sugar), and melatonin (which helps regulate sleep) have a direct impact on how we feel and function.

Picture a stressful day that just won't end. Your cortisol levels stay high, interfering with sleep, weakening immunity, and possibly leading to weight gain. Insulin, on the other hand, keeps blood sugar stable, but when imbalanced, it can lead to blood sugar crashes, leaving you irritable, tired, or craving unhealthy foods. Aim for consistent sleep; balanced meals with complex carbs, proteins, and healthy fats; and regular movement to support your endocrine system. These habits help keep your hormones steady, boosting energy and improving mood.

Your digestive system—from mouth to intestines—breaks

down food, absorbs nutrients, and eliminates waste. However, due to its close ties with the microbiome and nervous system, it's also a central player in the mind-body connection.

If you've ever experienced an upset stomach during a period of intense stress, you're already familiar with this connection. Stress can disrupt the digestive process, leading to acid reflux, bloating, or even irritable bowel syndrome (IBS). Supporting digestion through mindful eating, hydration, and fiber-rich foods does more than aid nutrient absorption—it also reduces stress on the gut, boosting both physical and emotional well-being.

So, in practical terms, how do we make the mind-body connection work in our favor?

Influencing the mind-body axis is achieved by being intentionally conscious of the impact of negative or positive thoughts on our health. As mentioned, stress can produce adrenaline and cortisol, two hormones associated with the fight-or-flight response. While this response can be useful in short-term emergencies, prolonged stress leads to elevated hormone levels that can damage our physical and psychological health.

Delving into the vast world of medicine highlights the cultural differences of how we approach healthcare. While Western medicine focuses on treating symptoms and individual parts of the body, it's often done without considering the interconnectedness of the being. Traditional healthcare practices such as Ayurveda or traditional Chinese medicine approach health holistically. They consider the scientific, energetic (chakras or qi), emotional, and even seasonal factors when investigating health issues. Interestingly, Western medicine is shifting from its narrow focus on isolated specifics toward a more integrated approach that also recognizes the importance of interconnectedness. Despite this shift, most Western healthcare providers still emphasize specialization, attributing illnesses to specific organs or systems. As the data suggests, incorporating a comprehensive approach to your mind-body axis can make a tangible improvement in your health. While this makes logical sense, it's admittedly a bit hard to quantify.

To truly thrive in your Second Prime, cultivating a compassionate, attuned, and coherent relationship with your body is essential. If you're willing to listen, your body holds a wealth of information, reflecting the impacts of your thoughts, lifestyle, and emotions. How often do we pause to listen without judgment and offer ourselves care? We usually overlook the signals our bodies are trying to communicate to us; I am guilty of this willful ignorance for sure. The connection you build with your body shapes how you care for yourself, influencing every facet of your being. The inner dialogue you engage in—whether loving or critical—deeply affects your overall well-being. As we age, self-compassion becomes both a practice and a powerful form of self-care.

Are you living your aligned truth? Or does your body tell a different story? Your physical state can reveal signals of this connection or disconnection. Some signals are subtle, others not so much. Paying attention to your body's signals provides a personalized road map to creating the life you want.

In my thirties and forties, I found myself in moments of piercing clarity, often followed by waves of intense dread. For nearly two decades, I sat in corporate meetings, feeling overwhelmed and anxious, my heart racing, a subtle panic echoing in my chest. Beneath it all, there was a nagging sense of fraudulence, always going back to the same question, *What am I doing here?* I had a feeling that I was wearing someone else's skin. My entire physiological system was on high alert, signaling that I was disconnected from my true self. Even when writing about it now, my heart rate starts to quicken, and I am transported back to the panic room that was my body. My body, wise and persistent, was trying to get my attention. But I kept ignoring it. So, why wasn't I listening?

What force kept me trapped, pushing me further from who I was and who I wanted to become?

During an especially difficult period at work, I lost my voice—literally. Recurrent bouts of laryngitis silenced me completely, and I now see it as my body's way of screaming for change. By silencing my voice, it was pointing to an undeniable truth: I was in the wrong place, living a life misaligned with my values. In that toxic work environment, I felt powerless and invisible, voiceless both physically and metaphorically. Yet despite recognizing the need for change and the value of alignment, my thoughts spiraled back to my family and financial responsibilities. I felt trapped by my circumstances, leaving me in a state of depletion and paralysis.

I stayed boxed in, confined by a story I kept telling myself: that safety meant staying put, no matter how deep the dissatisfaction. Instead of listening to my inner voice and honoring the discontent that surfaced time and again, I succumbed to self-imposed restrictions. I rationalized my choices, convincing myself that I was fine in this box I had built. But I was not fine, and it was a lie I told myself daily—a story of settling for less. In truth, I had abandoned my authenticity, accepting a life where I settled, settled, and settled some more.

Although my box felt familiar and it allowed me to provide for my family, it was soul-sucking; I began to feel the oppression of being silenced. Change became necessary when I realized I was making myself physically sick. At the time, I thought the connection was just anecdotal or a hunch. But now, research has revealed that a mismatch between your job and your true self can have negative effects on your health. A study from the Harvard T.H. Chan School of Public Health discovered that individuals who were dissatisfied with their employment had a 25 percent increased risk of coronary heart disease compared to those who felt happy and satisfied in their careers.

What's particularly fascinating is how this research validates what our bodies have been telling us all along. A 2023 longitudinal study found that people who reported feeling trapped in their careers showed measurably higher levels of inflammatory markers—the same markers associated with accelerated aging. But here's the hopeful part: When participants made changes to align their work with their values, these biological markers began to reverse within months. Our bodies aren't just sending us messages; they're offering us a road map to vitality.

Living out of alignment in our Second Prime isn't just an emotional burden. It creates a cascade of physiological responses that can fundamentally alter how we age. Our bodies carry the weight of our choices, not just as fleeting sensations, but as deeply embedded patterns that shape our physical experience of life. When we live misaligned from our true nature, our bodies respond with unmistakable clarity. Chronic tension becomes our constant companion, not just as temporary discomfort, but as a sustained pattern that reshapes our posture and movement. Our breathing becomes shallow, reducing oxygen flow to our tissues and accelerating cellular aging.

Our digestive system—that remarkable interpreter of our lived experience—begins to protest, leading to chronic inflammation that can accelerate the aging process. I've witnessed this transformation in my own body during those years of corporate misalignment. The persistent knot in my stomach during meetings wasn't just anxiety; it was my body's wisdom speaking through my vagus nerve, the superhighway of communication between gut and brain. Recent research has revealed that this nerve plays a crucial role in our aging process, influencing everything from inflammation levels to cellular repair.

When we ignore its signals, we're not just dismissing temporary discomfort; we're overriding one of our body's most sophisticated guidance systems. The Second Prime arrives with its own profound wisdom: We've reached a stage where we can no longer afford to ignore these signals. Our bodies have accumulated decades of insight, and they're demanding to be heard. That persistent shoulder pain isn't random. It might be the physical manifestation of carrying responsibilities that no longer serve our deepest purpose. The chronic digestive issues aren't merely about diet. They could be our body's protest against situations and relationships that don't nourish our true nature.

The science is unequivocal: Chronic misalignment triggers a stress response that floods our system with cortisol, increasing inflammation and accelerating cellular aging. A groundbreaking study from the *Journal of Aging Research* found that individuals who reported living in alignment with their values showed remarkably different biological markers than those who didn't. Their telomeres (protective ends on our chromosomes that influence how we age) were measurably longer, suggesting a slower aging process at the cellular level. Yet our bodies possess an extraordinary capacity for renewal when we finally listen. Within weeks of making changes that honor our true nature, measurable shifts begin to occur. Blood pressure normalizes, inflammation markers decrease, and even our sleep patterns improve. One participant in a recent study captured this transformation perfectly: "It felt like my body let out a breath it had been holding for twenty years."

Understanding these biological realities of alignment isn't just theoretical. It opens the door to practical tools for transformation. This is where the practice of mindsight becomes invaluable. Mindsight, as described by Dr. Dan Siegel, is a powerful tool for cultivating a deeper connection with our inner world. Defined as a focused attention that allows us to see the internal workings of our mind, mindsight enables us to observe our thoughts and emotions without judgment, creating a vital space between feeling and reaction. This conscious awareness disrupts the automatic responses we often fall into, allowing for a gentler, more compassionate approach to our inner dialogue. In this way, mindsight becomes a gateway to understanding and transforming how we relate to ourselves.

One of the most profound effects of mindsight is its impact on the mind-body axis. By practicing nonjudgmental observation of our thoughts, we reduce the impact of chronic stress and foster alignment—a state in which our mental, emotional, and physical responses are harmonized. Mindsight enables us to approach emotions like stress or frustration with curiosity rather than resistance, reducing the physiological responses that often accompany these emotions, such as elevated cortisol levels, inflammation, and muscle tension. This shift directly benefits the body by lowering stress responses, easing the strain on immune functions, and creating a sense of inner coherence, which leads to greater physical resilience.

Through the practice of mindsight, we can reframe unkind self-talk, moving from automatic criticism to compassionate awareness. Studies have shown that positive self-talk and emotional regulation directly influence the brain's neuroplasticity—the ability to reorganize and create new neural pathways. When we replace habitual self-criticism with supportive inner dialogue, mindsight helps retrain our brains to respond with kindness, reducing reactivity and building resilience. This process is particularly impactful as it gradually rewires our neural pathways, supporting healthier emotional and physiological responses, including decreased inflammation and a more balanced hormonal state.

Over time, mindsight also enhances coherence within the autonomic nervous system, regulating heart, digestion, and respiratory rates. A coherent nervous system is more adaptable and able to shift smoothly between relaxation and action in response to life's demands. This adaptability supports physical health and emotional flexibility, allowing us to recover more quickly from stressors and maintain emotional stability. Research even indicates that coherence within the heart-brain connection, often referred to as heart rate variability (HRV), improves with practices that foster mindfulness and self-compassion. A high HRV is associated with greater resilience and a reduced risk of cardiovascular disease, reflecting the profound impact of mental coherence on physical health.

In essence, mindsight cultivates a state of alignment and coherence that fosters well-being across all levels of the mind-body axis. When our inner dialogue is compassionate and our emotions are processed with awareness, the body follows suit, responding with reduced inflammation, improved immunity, and enhanced resilience. By developing this mindful relationship with ourselves, we create a feedback loop where mental clarity and physical health reinforce one another, forming a foundation for a more resilient, harmonious, and fulfilling life.

This conscious awareness becomes particularly powerful in our Second Prime, when we've accumulated enough life experience to recognize our patterns yet still have the vitality to reshape them. Recent neuroscience research reveals that our brains retain remarkable plasticity well into our sixties and seventies. Each time we pause to observe our thoughts rather than react to them, we're literally rewiring our neural pathways, creating new possibilities for how we experience our lives.

Following your inconvenient dream is a large component of alignment because having a purpose has been shown to positively impact biological markers for health on the mind-body axis. A study published in the journal *Health Psychology* found that having a purpose in life is associated with lower cortisol levels, which may reduce the risk of heart disease, depression, and other health concerns.

I hope you find this information as powerful as I do. Understanding the intricate dynamics between our conscious and unconscious thoughts, cognitive processes, and physical health is truly inspiring. While certain aspects of our biology are inherited, our mindset and behaviors offer a profound way to influence our well-being. By exploring the mechanisms that connect mind and body, we open new possibilities for cultivating resilience, health, and fulfillment. This deeper awareness is an investment in a healthier, more aligned future.

Notice the theme of alignment. Your subconscious knows what your conscious mind may deny. Your subconscious knows when you're in alignment with your true self. Recent advancements in the fields of psychology and physiology have helped us better understand the power of this connection. For our bodies to heal naturally, it's essential to maintain a harmonious whole-body relationship. Disruptions to this balance can lead to psychological and physical distress. Thoughts, emotions, hormones, neurotransmitters, and physiological responses are all interconnected.

Living on purpose is a choice. You can choose to live reactively, letting circumstances dictate your path, or proactively, pursuing what gives your life meaning. The power to determine your destiny is in your hands. What will you choose? To live purposefully or drift aimlessly?

Living in accordance with our inner selves fosters greater fulfillment and happiness.

Your physical and psychological well-being during your Second Prime depends on your courage to take chances and step out of the patterns you've been clinging to out of fear or habit. So, ask yourself: *What is holding me back? What signals has my mind-body connection been sending that I've brushed aside?* Perhaps it's the tension in your shoulders, the tightness in your chest, or the nagging sense that you're not living fully. These are not just discomforts to ignore—they're messages from your body, calling for change, urging you to move toward alignment and purpose.

Your Second Prime is your chance to listen deeply. This phase of life is a gift, an invitation to release those longings quietly waiting for expression. It's the perfect time to pursue your passions, to tap into what brings you alive. Remember, your future self is asking you to take action now—to care for the person you're becoming by nurturing the body and mind that will carry you there.

As you practice these steps, remember that alignment isn't achieved overnight. Often, it's more about bringing yourself back to your center, an ongoing return to self. It's a journey, one step at a time, toward a life that feels sincerely yours. By bringing your mind, body, and spirit into harmony, you create the conditions for thriving in your Second Prime. Listen deeply, act boldly, and let each small act of alignment be a promise to your future self.

While the science of mind-body alignment is complex, the path to living it is beautifully simple, though not always easy. It begins with small, conscious choices to honor what your body is telling you.

Challenge: Bring Yourself into Alignment

This week, commit to strengthening the dialogue between your mind and body. Here are four steps to help bring alignment into focus:

1. **Mindful Body Check-In:** Each morning, spend a few minutes quietly observing your body's sensations. Close your eyes, take a few deep breaths, and scan from head to toe. Notice any areas of tension, warmth, or discomfort without

judgment. Reflect on what these sensations might be trying to tell you. Is there a part of your life where you feel constrained or out of balance? Let these insights guide your intentions for the day.

2. **Practice Mindsight:** Throughout the day, practice observing your thoughts without reacting. When a critical or discouraging thought arises, pause. Imagine that thought as a passing cloud, simply moving through your mind. Acknowledge it without judgment, then reframe it with compassion. For example, if you catch yourself thinking, *I can't take that leap; it's too late for me,* try, *My Second Prime is exactly the right time for this adventure. I am allowed to grow and explore.*

3. **Daily Expression of Alignment:** Take one small action that brings you closer to alignment with your true self each day. This could be as simple as saying no to something that doesn't serve you, setting aside time for a passion project, or having an honest conversation with someone you trust. Notice how even the smallest step toward alignment feels in your body and heart. How does it impact your energy, outlook, and inner dialogue?

4. **Consider Keeping a Body Wisdom Journal:** Track these subtle signals and their meanings. One study participant in her mid-fifties discovered that her chronic neck pain disappeared completely within weeks of leaving a toxic work environment—not because the physical demands changed, but because she finally honored what her body had been trying to tell her for years. Your body's messages aren't just random symptoms; they're an intelligent guidance system pointing you toward your most aligned life.

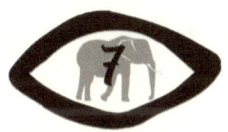

The Chemistry of Calm: From Hippie Wisdom to Harvard Research

Spirituality lives in the spaces between breaths, in those quiet moments when we pause long enough to hear the whispers of our own wisdom. Like many of us in our Second Prime, I've learned that this inner landscape holds secrets that science is only beginning to understand. It is a fascinating confluence of ancient wisdom and modern discovery that shapes not just our minds but also the very expression of our DNA.

In my case, I was raised by hippies, although "raised" might be too strong a word. My parents were young, wide-eyed wanderers of the late sixties who embraced the countercultural ethos in all its messy glory . . . and I was their hippie baby. Barefoot and free, in a little smocked dress (a style I still hold a fondness for), my sun-streaked hair wild and flowing, I was a true free-range child. Sweet pea flowers and sage are powerful scents of my childhood, mingling with the earthy smell of rain-soaked garden soil and sun-warmed grass. Those early years were untamed, a kaleidoscope of nature and open skies, where structure was as elusive as the morning mist, and running away from our cranky goose was the norm.

Ah, the pearls from my turbulent childhood! Thanks to loads of therapy, I now see the unexpected gifts those years offered. I vividly remember my dad and his girlfriend trying to teach me how to meditate—I must have been five or six. They were avid meditators, and our home was filled with their daily rituals of meditation and yoga. I'd sit on the floor, legs crossed, eyes closed, chanting "ohm" and counting breaths. My youthful energy rebelled against the stillness; it took every ounce of willpower not to jump up and race around the room.

Like so many of us, I have mixed emotions and scattered memories of my early childhood—a collection of impressions rather than an organized narrative. Those lessons in stillness, though challenging for a child bursting with energy, planted seeds that would later bloom into something profound. What I didn't understand then—what was not fully appreciated by science—was how these practices would eventually be validated by clinical research, revealing the extraordinary power of meditation to reshape not just our thoughts, but the very structure of our brains and the expression of our genes.

Our family life was wild, full of color but largely devoid of structure or stability. Security was an elusive concept; we lived moment to moment, my fractured family unit doing the best they could with what they had. Limited resources, youthful ideals, and well-meaning but often unconventional thoughts came together in a bright, but sometimes chaotic, family creation. They were simply trying to carve out a unique way, navigating the world with more heart than plan.

This unconventional beginning, though challenging, held a silver lining for me. What I lacked as a child, I was driven to seek as an adult. My wayward start instilled in me a deep need to cultivate calmness and find my own steady center. My mother gained confidence over the years, our lives grew more stable, and I'm forever grateful for her bravery and strength. Yet, those early years of unpredictability left an indelible mark that fueled my dedication to building a peaceful, centered inner world—a sanctuary of stillness and resilience. Looking back, I see both the beauty and the challenges of those years, the freedom and the uncertainty woven together. There's a sense of tenderness in remembering it now, acknowledging both the gifts and the gaps in my childhood. It's a complex memory, and yet, in its own way, it shaped the roots of who I am today.

The years of chaos revealed to me, in stark clarity, that I wanted and needed a personal oasis of harmony that I could reach at any time, regardless of my physical location. Determined to break free from the "crazy" I'd grown up with, I sought out therapy as soon as I could. The minute I had my first job with insurance, I found a therapist who helped me learn how to create and protect my peace. It was one of the best decisions I've ever made. I wanted emotional clarity, to learn how to step back and view my feelings with gentle detachment when needed. Building that inner equanimity became my mission, knowing this skill would allow me to meet life's ups and downs with grace.

Mindfulness—that precious quality of present-moment awareness—exists at a fascinating intersection of science and lived experience. It's both a cornerstone of the mind-body connection we explored in our last chapter and something far more expansive: a way of moving through the world with heightened awareness, a practice that grounds us in the present moment, and a state of being that transforms how we experience our lives. Think of mindfulness as a prism through which we experience reality, each facet offering a different dimension of awareness. In one moment, it's the practiced focus that notices tension creeping into our shoulders as we read emails. In another, it's the spontaneous appreciation of warm sunlight dancing across our couch when we enjoy our morning coffee. It's both the formal meditation practice where we sit in silence and the informal practice of bringing full attention to washing dishes or listening to a loved one speak.

This multidimensional nature of mindfulness makes it uniquely powerful in our Second Prime journey. When we cultivate mindfulness, we're not just engaging in a mental exercise; we're activating intricate networks of neural pathways that connect our thoughts, emotions, and physical sensations.

At the Lazar Lab for Meditation Research at Massachusetts General Hospital and Harvard Medical School, researchers have watched in amazement as meditation reshapes the very architecture of our brains. Through advanced imaging studies, they've witnessed how this ancient practice lights up networks of neural pathways like stars coming alive in the evening sky. Pathways that orchestrate our attention, regulate our emotions, and heighten our awareness of the body's subtle signals. These findings mirror what I've felt in my own practice; that each moment of mindful attention is like dropping a pebble in a pond, sending ripples of transformation through every aspect of our being.

The evidence for these transformative effects isn't just anecdotal; it's written in the growing body of research that bridges ancient wisdom with modern science. Thousands of studies show that, consistent with the range of spiritual practices, meditation and mindfulness can usher in a profound sense of inner peace and strength, enhance our overall health, sharpen cognitive function, nurture loving relationships, and deepen our connection to both ourselves and others.

More than just abstract benefits, these are tangible shifts that reshape our daily experience of living. What makes this journey particularly meaningful in our Second Prime is how it aligns with our natural inclination toward deeper understanding and authentic living. We've moved beyond the need to prove ourselves to others; now we're answering a more profound call, which is the invitation to explore our inner landscape with the same curiosity and wonder we once reserved for external adventures. This stage of life offers us a unique vantage point where we can appreciate both the vastness of possibility and the precious promise of a full, integrated self.

Like an energetic fingerprint, spirituality is individual, personal, and unique to you. You need not have religious beliefs or worship a god to be deeply connected to your spirit. The path you create is shaped by your preferences and perspectives. Feeding your soul is a journey of self-discovery. It can involve multiple practices, from meditation, prayer, and mindfulness to soaking in nature's serenity, equine therapy, exercise, chanting, and more. Each approach offers its own doorway to deeper awareness, its own language for speaking to the soul.

But the story of meditation's transformative power reaches even deeper, into the very essence of our physical being. The science behind meditation reveals its profound impact on our cellular health, touching the subtle machinery that governs our aging process. Dr. Elizabeth Blackburn's Nobel Prize–winning research on telomeres (those delicate protective caps at the end of our chromosomes that influence aging) unveiled an extraordinary discovery. Regular meditation can help maintain telomere length, potentially slowing the cellular dance of time itself. In the quiet moments of our practice, as our breath flows like a gentle tide, we're not just finding peace, we're engaging in an intimate dialogue with our very DNA, whispering messages of renewal and resilience to every cell in our body.

As we reach our Second Prime and beyond, this deeper understanding of how we can nourish our spirit and soul impacts not only our health and well-being, but also fundamentally shapes how we age physiologically. At the Center for Healthy Minds at the University of Wisconsin–Madison, Dr. Richard Davidson and his team have spent decades mapping the meditation-transformed brain. Through their longitudinal studies, published in journals like *NeuroImage* and *Frontiers in Psychology*, they've documented something remarkable. The brain of a long-term meditator shows enhanced thickness in regions associated with attention, emotional regulation, and self-awareness. It's as if meditation acts like a gentle sculptor, gradually refining and strengthening the neural networks that support our emotional well-being and cognitive clarity. When I learned of these findings, I couldn't help but reflect on my own journey from those initial thirty-second meditation sessions to the deeper practice I maintain today, each moment of mindfulness leaving its subtle imprint on my brain's living architecture.

Creating a meditation practice is a highly personal journey, yet it doesn't need to be complicated or overwhelming. Begin by choosing rituals that resonate with your beliefs and lifestyle. These could be as simple as a few minutes of deep breathing, a daily prayer, or even a silent reflection on your intentions for the day. The essential part is to gradually commit to a small amount of time each day—whether it's one minute or ten—and grow this practice.

I've always loved a good self-challenge. I break things down into the smallest possible steps to avoid feeling overwhelmed or discouraged and build from there. When I began meditating again eleven years ago, I started with just thirty seconds twice a day. Back then, anxiety was my constant companion, and meditation offered a far more lasting comfort than any quick fix—a glass of wine, a binge on comfort food, or even anti-anxiety medication.

In those tiny increments of stillness, I found something invaluable: a sense of peace that came from within, not from anything external. What I didn't understand then—but have come to appreciate deeply through both experience and scientific discovery—is how these brief moments of stillness were literally reshaping my brain's chemical landscape. Each time I sat in meditation I was conducting an intricate cascade of neurotransmitters—the brain's messengers of well-being and balance.

This biological process begins subtly. As we settle into meditation, our brain starts to shift its chemical composition. Dopamine, our motivation messenger, begins to flow more freely, bringing with it a natural sense of focus and clarity that no amount of caffeine can replicate. Serotonin levels rise, easing the grip of anxiety and wrapping us in a blanket of emotional stability. Meanwhile, GABA—nature's own anti-anxiety compound—increases, helping to quiet the mental chatter that so often drowns out our inner wisdom. The beauty of this process lies in its cumulative effect.

Just as my practice grew from thirty seconds to longer periods, these neurological benefits compound over time. The brain's production of acetylcholine and glutamate increases, supporting not just our present peace but our future cognitive resilience—a gift particularly precious in our Second Prime. Even melatonin, our sleep regulator, responds to this practice, helping to establish the kind of deep, restorative rest that becomes more elusive as we age. What moves me most about this science is how it validates what ancient wisdom traditions have long known—these seemingly simple practices of stillness and breath awareness are anything but simple in their effects. When we meditate, we're not just calming our thoughts, we're actively participating in our brain's renewal. The lowering of stress hormones like cortisol creates space for something remarkable; the emergence of compounds like DMT— associated with creativity and spiritual awareness—reminding us that our capacity for growth and insight doesn't diminish with age. Instead, it deepens.

This commitment to cultivating a calm strength in our Second Prime becomes even more critical as this time in our life often deals us the highest number of challenges. The inner peace we build impacts every facet of our well-being, from mental health to physical vitality to relationships. With each experience, we gain insight and resilience, allowing us to navigate this stage of life with joy, clarity, and intention. To live joyfully, it's essential to cultivate a loving, fearless relationship with oneself, and exploring our inner emotions is a crucial part of that journey. Our mental and emotional health are every bit as vital as our physical well-being, and spirituality offers a profound pathway to understanding our deeper selves.

Self-love, after all, is the foundation of loving others. Through meaningful spiritual practices, we can learn to see ourselves with greater compassion and acceptance, enabling us to share more of our love and light with those around us. This journey is medicine for the spirit.

Creating a personal oasis—a space where you feel calm and grounded in the middle of life's chaos—isn't just a practice; it's a gift to yourself that can unlock incredible growth. It builds inner strength, a quiet resilience that you might not even realize is there until life inevitably throws its curveballs. When we nurture this place of calm within, we're not just coping; we're cultivating a deep-rooted power that keeps us steady, no matter how the world shifts around us. Start small, trust the process, and watch how even the tiniest commitment to yourself can ripple through every part of your life.

For those who find meditation daunting or challenging, consider that your mind's constant flow of thoughts is not a flaw but a feature. The mind is dynamic by design, generating thoughts as naturally as the heart beats. The goal of meditation is not to silence the mind but to observe these thoughts without attachment, to witness rather than react. This process helps you cultivate stability that can be sustained throughout the day. Start by focusing on a single point of awareness—your breath, a mantra, or even a gentle sound in your environment. Begin with just one minute each day and gradually increase as it feels comfortable. Meditation is called a practice because it is a journey, not a destination. Embrace it as an act of self-kindness, a chance to greet each thought with curiosity rather than judgment.

If you're new to meditation or have tried to create a practice and it's been elusive, *beditation*—meditating right from the
comfort of bed—might be a gentle way to ease into it. Before the
demands of the day take hold, try placing your earbuds in as soon
as you wake up and listening to a guided meditation. Lying in
bed, relaxed and open, allows you to start your day from a place
of calm intention. Even a few minutes of beditation can help set
the tone for your day, grounding you in peace before stepping into
the world.

Similarly, *yoga nidra*, also known as yogic sleep, is a practical
entry point for those who struggle with traditional meditation.
Practiced while lying down, this guided meditation takes you
through stages of body awareness, breath control, and visualiza-
tion, guiding you toward deep relaxation without falling asleep.
Yoga nidra has been shown to reduce stress, improve sleep quality,
and even alter brain wave patterns, helping you access a calm,
meditative state with minimal effort. It's an ideal way to experience the benefits of meditation, especially if you're seeking a
gentler practice.

Both beditation and yoga nidra meet you where you are—
allowing you to cultivate mindfulness in the most relaxed state
possible. Whether in bed, lying on a yoga mat, or even in a comfortable chair, these approaches remind us that meditation is about
creating moments of awareness, not a blank mind. These practices
allow you to start slowly, building a foundation of mindfulness and
self-acceptance that can become the cornerstone of your practice
in your Second Prime.

Spirituality is where we can search for inner peace, tran-
scending the labels and roles that often divide us. It speaks to the
universal human yearning for the sacred—a search for meaning,
purpose, and connection with something greater than ourselves.
Whether we find that connection in a higher self, God, universal

energy, or simply in a shared community, spirituality has a powerful way of grounding us and guiding us through life's complexities. Embracing a spiritual practice isn't just about belief; it's a commitment that profoundly benefits mind, body, and soul. Studies affirm that spiritual practices bring tangible physiological and psychological benefits, irrespective of age or religious beliefs.

One extraordinary finding is that meditation has been scientifically shown to increase the thickness of gray matter in the brain, an effect observed even in later stages of life. This increase in gray matter, which is responsible for processing information, decision-making, memory, and emotions, demonstrates that meditation can help keep our brains sharp as we age. By nurturing gray matter, meditation bolsters our capacity for higher cognitive functions like memory, language, and emotional regulation. In a genuine sense, spiritual practices like meditation can support brain health and resilience, giving us tools to age with clarity and vitality.

The science behind meditation is equally fascinating. This inward journey doesn't just quiet the mind; it has powerful effects on the body, including our genes. Here's where epigenetics comes into play. *Epigenetics* is the study of how our behaviors and environment can change how our genes work. Unlike genetic changes, these modifications do not alter the DNA sequence but can still profoundly affect gene expression—turning specific genes on or off. Research shows that meditation, mindfulness, and even practices like gratitude can influence gene expression, promoting genes that help manage stress, boost immunity, and even slow down cellular aging.

So, how does this work? When we meditate, we activate the parasympathetic nervous system, our body's relaxation response. This shift reduces neurotransmitters like cortisol and increases beneficial neurotransmitters such as serotonin. Over time, regular meditation can lead to beneficial epigenetic changes—essentially reprogramming our body's responses to stress. This means that through a committed meditation and mindfulness practice, you are empowering your body to respond to life with resilience rather than reactivity.

Imagine each meditation session as a small yet profound act of nurturing your genetic potential. You're engaging in an inner dialogue with your cells, guiding them toward health and longevity. The way we live—especially the ways we choose to slow down and tune in—literally has the power to reshape our biology.

Countless studies confirm that those who adopt a spiritual practice experience heightened compassion, better stress management, improved social connections, and increased purpose in life, all skills vital for us Second Primers. We benefit from more compassion and less judgment toward others as well as more inner kindness. Aging with intention is a powerful act of courage, and self-compassion is a game-changing skill.

Additionally, research has revealed that meditation and mindfulness practices can lead to longer lifespans and improved physical health by reducing stress levels. Just as maintaining a healthy diet and exercise balance contributes to overall physical wellness, spirituality is equally impactful for our mental and emotional well-being. Taking time for solitude and reflection can awaken creativity, ignite inspiration, and facilitate a stronger connection with the greater good all around us. Understanding these benefits is one thing; creating a sustainable practice is another.

Challenge: Personal Time

This challenge is about building your own sanctuary of stillness, starting exactly where you are. Start your day with ease by waking up twenty minutes early and dedicating this time to a simple morning spiritual practice. To center yourself before the demands of the day set in, try a gentle meditation practice right from the comfort of your bed—it's time for some beditation! This simple, intentional ritual can transform how you engage with the world, infusing each day with calm and clarity.

1. **Set Your Intention:** Begin with a clear intention. Think about what you hope to gain from this practice—perhaps a sense of peace, focus, or a deeper connection to yourself. Repeating this intention silently, or even writing it down the night before, can make your practice more purposeful.

2. **Embrace Silence and Stillness:** As you wake, lie quietly before checking your phone or diving into tasks. Place your hands on your heart or belly and breathe deeply, focusing on each breath. Allow your mind to soften and release any urgency to think, plan, or worry. Just be.

3. **Mindful Breathing:** Slowly shift your attention to your breath. Inhale deeply for a count of four, hold for four, and exhale for six. Notice the rhythm, feel each breath move through your body, and ground yourself in this simple act of breathing.

4. **Express Gratitude:** Conclude with gratitude by thinking of three things you're thankful for—this can be as simple as appreciating a good night's rest, the gift of a new day, or the support of loved ones.

5. **Reflect on Your Routine:** If you already have a spiritual practice, ask yourself: *Has it become routine? Am I simply going through the motions?* Consider adding variety to your ritual—a few minutes of journaling, a new mantra, or a different breathing exercise. Small adjustments can reignite a deeper sense of presence and connection.

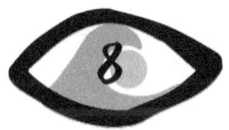

Softening into Strength: The Science of Emotional Mastery

In our Second Prime, we're entering a phase of life ripe with new potential—not just in our careers or social roles, but in our ability to nurture our inner lives and connections to others. Emotional intelligence, generosity, and gratitude are powerful tools that don't just elevate our minds and spirits but impact our physical health and resilience. This journey through the soft skills of wisdom and emotional awareness offers us a path to well-being and fulfillment that grows more robust with age.

At its core, *emotional intelligence* (EI) is the ability to understand and manage our emotions, recognize the emotions of others, and use this insight to guide our interactions and decisions. For years, society viewed EI as a nice-to-have, a secondary trait to hard skills like logic or analytical reasoning. However, new research shows that EI is vital for innovation, adaptability, and effective leadership, especially as we mature. Studies from Carstensen and colleagues reveal that emotional awareness increases with age, helping us better manage our feelings and cultivate a more profound empathy for others. This growing self-awareness is crucial in our Second Prime, where challenges and opportunities often require more thoughtful, emotionally nuanced responses.

To illustrate this development, consider a situation that could be familiar to many of us: Imagine someone accidentally bumps into you, causing you to stumble and drop the ice cream cone you are carrying onto your shirt. How might various stages of life handle this, and what's going on inside each one?

- **A Toddler** might burst into tears, immediately expressing disappointment and shock. Lacking the words or self-awareness to process complex emotions, they respond in the most direct way possible. Internally, the toddler's brain is still developing its emotional regulation abilities, and the amygdala—the brain's fight-or-flight center—reacts quickly to sudden stimuli, triggering a flood of stress hormones like cortisol. Without developed neural pathways for calming responses, toddlers often express their emotions as they feel them—unfiltered and unrestrained.

- **A Teenager** might respond with irritation or frustration, perhaps vocalizing their irritation or storming off. Internally, they are just beginning to develop an understanding of other people's perspectives, but powerful emotions still overshadow their ability to empathize. Physiologically, teenagers experience elevated dopamine levels in their brains, enhancing the intensity of experiences and feelings. As the prefrontal cortex—responsible for impulse control and long-term reasoning—is still maturing, teenagers may feel compelled to express their frustration outwardly rather than manage it internally. This stage is a complex balancing act of growing empathy and robust physiological responses that drive high emotional reactivity.

- **A Thirtysomething** might feel a mix of embarrassment and frustration. Social dynamics and perception are powerful at this age, making them keenly aware of how others see them. They might feel the impulse to react but try to maintain composure, especially in public. Physiologically, they have greater control over the amygdala's response and more developed pathways in the prefrontal cortex to help moderate emotions. However, stress responses like a slight spike in adrenaline might still occur, elevating heart rate and some-times intensifying their embarrassment. Their awareness of others' perceptions can make regulating their emotions challenging, as the desire to save face competes with their reaction to the accident.

- **A Second Primer** may manage this situation with perspec-tive and grace. They might offer a calm smile, reassuring the person who caused the fumble and perhaps even laughing it off to diffuse any tension. At this stage, they have a rich library of life experiences, including moments like this, and have likely learned that minor inconveniences don't need to escalate into larger problems.

- **A Senior with Decades of Wisdom** might respond simi-larly to someone in their Second Prime but with even more measured calm and empathy. With a deep understanding of life's unpredictability and an even more tempered response to minor inconveniences, they might brush off the incident with a warm smile and turn the moment into an opportu-nity for gentle humor. Internally, their brain's response to stress is further reduced as life experience has refined their stress-management techniques.

Research shows that older adults tend to have lower cortisol responses to daily stressors, indicating an overall increased resili-ence. They've developed an ability to interpret such situations not as nuisances but as small, teachable moments of kindness and understanding. This level of emotional intelligence highlights the profound maturity that comes with age, where they choose responses that align with their values of compassion and patience.

But beneath these seemingly simple responses lies a fascinating cascade of neurological processes that transforms a mere accident into an opportunity for connection. In that split second when ice cream meets clothing, the Second Primer's brain has developed what neuroscientists call *cognitive empathy networks*. These intricate neural pathways allow them to instantly recognize and resonate with the mortification likely flooding through the person who bumped into them, their own discomfort becoming secondary to the shared human experience unfolding in this public space.

While younger brains might flood with cortisol and adrenaline, triggering that instinctive fight-or-flight response, the Second Primer's brain has developed a more nuanced chemical ballet. Research from the Stanford Center on Longevity reveals that as we age, our brains become better at integrating emotional and rational thinking. The neural pathways between emotional centers and decision-making regions become more efficiently connected, allowing for what we might call emotional wisdom—the ability to process complex social situations with both heart and mind engaged simultaneously.

In this moment, they might notice their heart rate increase slightly, but rather than this physiological response escalating into stress, it becomes background noise to a more profound awareness. Their experienced neural networks are already crafting a response that will ease everyone's tension, perhaps sharing a story about their own similar mishap from years ago. They notice the stranger's trembling hands as they offer napkins, the concerned glances from others nearby, and their own soiled clothes, all while maintaining a presence that transforms discomfort into connection.

This isn't just emotional intelligence. It's emotional artistry, painted with brushstrokes of neuroplasticity and lived experience. Their brain's prefrontal cortex, now at peak maturity, works in harmony with an experienced amygdala to recognize that this situation isn't a threat but rather an opportunity for human connection. The parasympathetic nervous system—the rest-and-digest response—maintains calm, minimizing the release of corti-sol and allowing them to regulate their reaction effectively.

What's occurring isn't simply the absence of stress. It's the presence of something far more sophisticated: a well-orches-trated symphony of neurotransmitters and neural pathways that have learned to dance together in service of something greater than self-preservation. It's the biological foundation of wisdom, expressed through a smile that says, *We're all human, and this moment, too, shall become a story worth telling.*

This is the gift of the Second Prime, the ability to transform what could be a moment of tension into one of genuine human connection backed by the fascinating science of our evolving emo-tional capabilities. It's a reminder that our capacity for empathy and understanding doesn't diminish with age but rather deepens, enriched by both lived experience and the remarkable adaptability of our evolving brains.

This progression underscores what it means to grow into emo-tional intelligence over time. In our Second Prime, we've learned that our reactions are within our control, and we choose responses that foster connection, respect, and understanding. These small moments reveal the depth of our emotional growth, allowing us to approach even challenging situations with empathy and composure.

Standing at the midpoint of life offers us a unique vantage point. We can look backward with clarity, tracing the many choices that brought us here, while forward lies a landscape visible only through the imprecise telescope of hope . . . and maybe a bit of fear. Around us walk the living prophecies—those who've mastered the alchemy of years, transmuting time into wisdom, messengers who tell us aging can be done well. And others who've let their days calcify into bitter monuments to what might have been. In their faces, we read our possible futures, showing us that how we engage with our remaining years determines whether we continue to evolve or slowly ossify into monuments to our past selves.

Think of that uncle or family friend at family gatherings (we all have one) who's transformed grumpiness into an art form or that neighbor who's practicing for their future role as the self-appointed lawn enforcement officer. These aren't just characters in life's grand comedy. They're glimpses into potential futures, gentle reminders of the choices that lie ahead on our own journey from midlife to what's next.

The path before us isn't marked by bitter or better. It's illuminated by the choices we make in these middle years, where each day offers a fresh page in our unfolding story. These chapters we're writing now aren't about avoiding aging's challenges but about choosing how we'll meet them—with resistance that drains our spirit or with wisdom that transforms each year into an opportunity for deeper understanding and richer living. It's in catching ourselves in those small moments, when we feel the urge to perfect our own version of the disapproving "tsk" or find ourselves rehearsing that theatrical throat-clearing that seems to come standard issue with advanced years. These moments of recognition arrive like little cosmic nudges, asking us, *Which way am I leaning?*

The beauty lies in realizing we don't have to wait for our Second Prime to choose our path. Every eyeroll at slower shoppers, every muttered commentary about "kids these days," every temptation to become the spatial awareness challenger in the grocery store—these are all early choreography for the dance we'll eventually perform. Will we practice the steps of grace and understanding or perfect the shuffle of perpetual disapproval?

This awareness is perhaps one of the most valuable gifts of midlife—the recognition that while we can't control time's forward march, we can shape how it molds us. We're not just passive observers watching the preview of possible futures. We're the directors of our own becoming, choosing scene by scene whether we'll lean toward light or shadow.

After all, emotional intelligence isn't something that magically appears with gray hair, it's a skill we need to tend now, in these pivotal middle years. Each choice to respond with grace instead of grievance, each decision to drop the pettiness when someone is rude or lacks social skills, each moment of choosing connection over criticism becomes part of the foundation for who we'll become.

So perhaps the next time we encounter one of those colorful characters who've embraced their role as professional curmudgeons, we might offer a quiet thanks for the preview of what low evolutionary behavior looks like and choose, with both humor and intention, to navigate toward a different future. Because the journey from midlife to Second Prime isn't just about getting older; it's about growing into the kind of person who makes others want to grow older too.

Physiologically, with each life stage, the brain increasingly shifts from reactive (amygdala driven) responses to reflective (prefrontal cortex driven) responses. In early life, emotions are intense and often overwhelming, but we gain the neurological and experiential tools to manage these responses better as we grow. The ability to navigate life's inevitable bumps with emotional awareness is a gift that amplifies with age. Through it, we realize that emotional intelligence isn't just about controlling reactions but about nurturing understanding, compassion, and a sense of calm in ourselves and others.

One of the many components of EI is generosity, though not in the material sense. It's a generosity of spirit—the inclination to share time, attention, and empathy with others. A *Harvard Business Review* study found that leaders with high EI who cultivate generosity in their approach to themselves and others are more successful in driving innovation and managing complex, creative teams. In our Second Prime, generosity becomes less about accruing status and more about sharing our life's wisdom and energy. For instance, think about how listening intently to a friend or offering guidance to a younger colleague creates a ripple effect of goodwill and connection. These moments, rooted in generosity, bring joy to others, and strengthen our neural pathways for empathy and joy.

Similarly, gratitude is an active choice to recognize and celebrate the good in our lives. Science shows that when practiced regularly, gratitude enhances neural plasticity, promoting mental flexibility and resilience. It's more than an occasional "thank you." It's a consistent, intentional way of viewing the world that fosters a deep appreciation for what we have. Studies reveal that people in their midlife and later years who practice gratitude experience improved mental and physical health, including better cardiovascular function and lower stress levels. When we express gratitude, we activate areas in the brain associated with reward and empathy, creating a cycle that reinforces positive emotions and improves our overall outlook.

The benefits of emotional intelligence, generosity, and gratitude aren't confined to our minds—they profoundly affect our bodies through an intricate dance of neurochemistry that grows more nuanced as we age. At the heart of this chemical symphony is oxytocin, often called the bonding hormone or love hormone, though these playful nicknames barely scratch the surface of its remarkable influence on our well-being.

Research from the Max Planck Institute for Evolutionary Anthropology reveals that oxytocin does more than just make us feel warm and fuzzy—it's a sophisticated combination of social connection and physical health. When we engage in acts of kindness, from mentoring others to volunteering, our bodies release this powerful molecule that reduces blood pressure, promotes heart health, helps regulate our inflammatory responses, and supports immune function.

Fascinatingly, as we move through midlife our relationship with oxytocin evolves. Studies from the University of California, San Diego suggest that while our baseline oxytocin levels may gradually decrease, our sensitivity to its effects can increase, making those moments of connection and generosity even more potent. It's as if our bodies become more attuned to the chemistry of compassion, allowing us to derive greater benefit from smaller doses of this remarkable molecule.

Acts of kindness, it turns out, are like compound interest for our well-being—they accumulate over time, strengthening both the giver and receiver. Our emotional muscles grow stronger with use, helping us manage stress better and increasing resilience against age-related decline. Research with over 50,000 adults aged between fifty-one and sixty-one showed that those who practiced empathy and emotional generosity experienced improvements in their physical health, with elevated oxytocin levels playing a crucial role in this mind-body connection.

In our journey toward our Second Prime, these practices allow us to be softer and stronger—softer in our responses and stronger in our mental and physical resilience. Every act of kindness, every moment of genuine connection, becomes not just an emotional investment but also a biological tune-up, helping our bodies and minds age with greater grace and vitality.

This focus is essential, helping us build a foundation and find our path. But something beautiful happens as we move through life—our perspective expands. The *me* drive gradually gives way to a *we* drive. We start seeing our lives in the context of others' lives, thinking less about what's in it for us and more about how we can contribute. This shift isn't accidental; it's deeply rooted in our biology.

Humans have evolved as social creatures, with connections as essential to survival as food or shelter. Early humans lived in close-knit groups, relying on cooperation and mutual support to meet basic needs and ward off threats. Studies show that bonding behaviors, such as sharing resources, caring for others, and displaying empathy, were favored by natural selection. Those who connected with others—by forming alliances, sharing food, and cooperating—were more likely to survive, pass on their genes, and foster the continuation of their group.

Picture the raw vulnerability of a single human against the elements, predators, and the sheer magnitude of survival's daily demands. Now contrast this with the strength found in numbers—multiple sets of eyes scanning for danger, many hands sharing the burden of gathering food, countless minds pooling their knowledge to solve problems. In the unforgiving laboratory of evolution, isolation wasn't just uncomfortable—it was often fatal.

This biological imperative for connection runs so deep that even today, when our physical survival seems less immediately threatened, our bodies and minds react to social isolation as if facing a mortal danger. Without the web of support that comes from genuine human connection, tasks that seem simple on the surface become monumentally challenging. Who would watch our children while we work? Who would care for us when illness strikes? Who would share their knowledge, their resources, their strength when ours fail?

Beyond mere survival, these connections created something even more remarkable: communities capable of accumulating and sharing wisdom, supporting innovation, and nurturing the kind of emotional intelligence that transforms mere existence into a life worth living. In our modern world, where technology often creates an illusion of self-sufficiency, acknowledging our deep-seated need for human connection becomes not just wise but revolutionary.

Today, connection remains essential for our health and well-being. Our bodies release oxytocin in response to positive social interactions, deepening trust and affection between people. Oxytocin is known to reduce stress, lower blood pressure, and enhance feelings of empathy, reinforcing our sense of connection and safety. Additionally, neurotransmitters like dopamine are activated when we engage in social bonding, reinforcing behaviors that build relationships and strengthen community ties.

Neuroscience research has also uncovered that our brains are wired for empathy through a system called mirror neurons. When we observe others' emotions or actions, our mirror neurons fire like we are experiencing these feelings ourselves. This mirroring ability helps us understand others and strengthens our social bonds by creating a shared emotional experience, which we'll explore more in the next chapter.

As we move into our Second Prime, this shift toward a *we* mindset profoundly benefits us and those we support. By embracing connection, we contribute to a world where everyone feels seen and valued and finds a sense of belonging that nourishes our mental and physical health. This phase of life invites us to rediscover the joy of being part of something larger than ourselves, fulfilling an ancient human need for togetherness and purpose.

In many ways, EI is the foundation of generosity. By understanding others' needs and feelings, we naturally want to help, uplift, and support. Research reveals that this inclination isn't simply good for our inner being; it's good for the body. In a study at Carnegie Mellon, adults who practiced regular acts of kindness—whether by offering help, listening deeply, or simply showing compassion—saw measurable improvements in their physical health. Inflammation markers dropped, cellular health improved, and resilience to stress soared. Generosity, driven by empathy, sustains life in an authentic, tangible way.

Generosity doesn't need to be grand. One of my favorite personal traditions is tipping restroom workers in airports. Think about it; everyone wants a clean restroom, yet few truly see the workers who maintain these spaces. These individuals do essential work in an often thankless environment, keeping everything sanitary and pleasant. Giving them a tip, a warm smile, and a few words of appreciation can make a significant difference in their day—and it makes me feel connected to something more significant, a part of a community that values all contributions. I would love to see this become a movement, a small gesture of respect for people who deserve to feel valued for the crucial role they play. And we all know that a cleaner, kinder world begins with these small but deeply meaningful actions.

Here are other simple yet powerful ways to bring generosity into your daily life:

- **Offer Genuine Praise:** Lift someone's spirits by noticing their hard work or creativity.

- **Encourage Someone's Inconvenient Dream:** Cheer someone on in their unique pursuits, even if they defy practicality.

- **Be Fully Present:** Give your undivided attention, make eye contact, and actively listen.

- **Acknowledge Overlooked Roles:** Show respect and gratitude to individuals whose work supports all of us but often goes unseen.

Challenge: Cultivating Your EI

As we navigate our Second Prime, cultivating emotional intelligence becomes less a destination and more a daily practice: a gentle awakening to the subtle currents that shape our responses and connections. Like tending a garden, this practice requires patience, attention, and a willingness to nurture growth in unexpected places. Consider the following reflection points to see where you are on your journey.

- How often do I practice self-compassion and patience?
- Do I offer love or kindness to others without conditions?
- Am I connected to my community in meaningful ways?

No matter how you answered the questions, there is space to grow your wisdom and EI. The following practices cultivate an optimistic outlook, which is central to successful aging. They transform our mindset from scarcity to abundance, helping us recognize our place within a greater community of humanity. Over time, you'll notice that these acts of kindness build emotional resilience and rewire your brain for positivity.

By embracing these practices of ritual and reflection, we're not just aging; we're evolving into the kind of presence that makes the world a little warmer, a little wiser, and a little more connected. This is the art of growing not just older, but also deeper into our shared humanity.

- Begin your day by sending messages of love and appreciation to at least three individuals. Go through your contact list and keep spreading love throughout the year. By doing so, you will have made a positive impact worldwide.

- Start a daily gratitude journal or list three things you are grateful for in the morning and the evening. This will take less than one minute.

- Each day, find a small way to give. It could be a kind word, a small favor, or a quick message to brighten someone's day.

- End your day by noting three meaningful moments. Reflect on these to deepen your appreciation and reinforce an inner sense of abundance.

- Revisit your inconvenient dream and ask yourself how to incorporate a giving practice related to your goals.

Wired to Connect: From Mirror Neurons
to Belly Laughs

Picture this: You're laughing so hard with an old friend that your cheeks hurt, tears streaming down your face as you try (and fail) to catch your breath. Maybe you snort. These kinds of moments aren't just good for your soul; they're keeping you vibrant and healthy at a cellular level. Increasing our lifespan is worthwhile only if our quality of life remains high; few people wish for a long, miserable existence.

The quality versus quantity equation demands intentional, consistent upkeep. Creating a vision that marries longevity with vitality in our Second Prime becomes crucial. This stage invites us to commit to habits and choices that support our future well-being. While genetics, education, and socioeconomic status play roles in how we age, prioritizing a balanced diet, exercise, and quality healthcare are foundational. Avoiding harmful habits and practicing simple safety measures—like flossing, wearing seatbelts, and using helmets—also significantly impacts our longevity.

But one game-changer is often overlooked, one factor that profoundly affects our health, resilience, joy, and even lifespan: connection. Our innate need to feel connected is as essential as any other lifestyle factor. Living a purposeful life and nurturing meaningful relationships are foundational to reaching our fullest potential.

Let me share something fascinating about how we're wired. At our core, humans are social creatures designed for cooperation and collaboration, a trait that didn't emerge by chance but through the crucible of survival itself. Our ancient ancestors understood what modern science now confirms. Belonging isn't just nice to have; it is essential for survival. Those early human bands, huddled around flickering fires under vast starlit skies, knew that isolation meant vulnerability, while connection meant strength, safety, and the sweet probability of seeing another dawn.

The impact of loneliness extends far beyond just feeling disconnected. It reverberates through every cell in our bodies, influencing not just how long we live, but how well we live. When researchers began measuring the effects of social isolation, they discovered something startling—emotional loneliness triggers the same inflammatory response as physical injury. Our bodies, in their ancient wisdom, recognize isolation as a threat as real as any wound.

The numbers tell a compelling story. Studies show that chronic loneliness can increase the risk of premature death by up to 26 percent. But even modest social connections can boost survival rates by up to 50 percent. Think about that for a moment. The simple act of maintaining meaningful connections isn't just about having someone to call when we need help moving furniture; it's about fundamentally altering our biological trajectory.

While regular exercise can add three to five years to your life expectancy, maintaining strong social connections can add seven to nine years. Dr. David Sinclair's groundbreaking research reveals that strong social ties rival the impact of diet, exercise, and sleep in promoting healthy aging. But beyond mere survival, recent studies in quality of life metrics show something equally powerful. Socially connected individuals report 60 percent higher rates of daily joy, twice the level of perceived purpose, and significantly better cognitive function well into their later years.

In our Second Prime, building authentic connections while being mindful of digital distractions may be one of the most powerful steps we can take toward a long, healthy, and fulfilling life. Smartphones are engineered to capture our attention with the precision of an expert jeweler. Studies show that the average person touches their phone 2,617 times per day—and it's not because we lack willpower. Tech companies employ teams of neuroscientists and behavioral psychologists to design apps that trigger our brain's reward centers, creating what scientists call intermittent variable rewards—the same mechanism that makes slot machines so compelling.

Our brains are masterpieces of social engineering, literally wired for connection in ways we're just beginning to understand. When we engage in face-to-face conversation, our brains create profound patterns of connection. Mirror neurons—those specialized brain cells that fire both when we perform an action and when we watch others perform the same action—create an automatic, unconscious synchrony between people. These neural mimics help us share emotions, understand intentions, and feel what others feel. It's why you might find yourself tearing up when a friend shares a painful story, or why a genuine smile from across the room can lift your mood instantly.

This neural dance goes even deeper. Scientists call it *neural synchrony*: a phenomenon where two brains begin to mirror each other's patterns during genuine connection. Through subtle micro-signals—the lift of an eyebrow, a shift in tone, the language of posture—our brains create harmonies of connection that enhance everything from cognitive function to emotional resilience.

Digital interactions, by contrast, often create what researchers call *parasocial relationships*. These are one-sided connections where we feel we know someone intimately, yet they know nothing about us. Think about scrolling through a friend's carefully curated Instagram feed versus sitting across from them at coffee, hearing the catch in their voice as they share a difficult truth. The first gives us the illusion of connection; the second creates genuine neural and emotional resonance.

Yet here's where it gets interesting; digital connection isn't inherently empty. Studies show that synchronous digital interactions—like video calls where we can see facial expressions and hear voice modulation in real-time—activate many of the same neural pathways as in-person meetings. It's the asynchronous, passive consumption of others' lives that tends to leave us feeling oddly hollow, even as we convince ourselves we're staying connected.

Research shows that adults over forty-five are actually more susceptible to notification disruption than younger users, possibly because our brains process multiple streams of information differently as we mature. It's not a weakness; it's neuroscience. The average social media app triggers dopamine releases more frequently than any natural reward system in human history, and our brains haven't evolved to resist these sophisticated attention capturing techniques.

But here's the empowering part: Understanding this dynamic gives us back our agency. When we recognize these patterns not as personal failings but as predictable responses to carefully engineered stimuli, we can make conscious choices about our attention. Research shows that simply being aware of these design mechanisms reduces their power over us by up to 40 percent.

What's fortunate about our Second Prime is that we're uniquely positioned to navigate this digital landscape with the wisdom that only experience can bring. We remember the art of long conversations that meandered like garden paths, the subtle pleasure of reading a friend's mood through the tiniest shift in their voice, the way time seemed to suspend itself during moments of genuine connection.

Speaking of genuine connection, there's one form of interaction that bypasses all our digital defenses and taps directly into our shared humanity—laughter. While our phones might buzz with endless notifications, nothing quite compares to the authentic, unfiltered joy of a real laugh shared with someone we love.

When we think about laughter, our minds might first go to the uniquely human, such as the shared joke over coffee or the belly laughs at a friend's story. But nature holds a delightful secret. Laughter ripples through the mammalian world like a joyful current, connecting species in a symphony of shared emotion. Scientists have now documented laughter-like vocalizations in at least sixty-five species of mammals, from the obvious to the unexpected.

The cast of laughing creatures tells a story of joy's evolution. There's the familiar pant-laughing of chimpanzees, who share not just our DNA but our capacity for contagious giggles. Gorillas produce a throaty chuckle during play that's remarkably similar to our own. Orangutans engage in what researchers call play-panting, their version of shared mirth. Even our dogs—those masters of human connection—have their own laugh-like panting that's so powerful it can calm other dogs in shelters.

But perhaps most surprising are the smaller players in this joyful chorus. Rats—those clever survivors of urban landscapes—emit ultrasonic chirps of delight when tickled or during play. It's a sound we can't hear without special equipment but that speaks to the universality of joy. Even dolphins, with their complex social lives beneath the waves, share laugh-like vocalizations during social bonding.

What makes this shared heritage of happiness so profound isn't just its breadth across species but what it tells us about the fundamental nature of joy and connection. Laughter, in all its forms, serves as a bridge between individuals, a signal of safety, play, and belonging that transcends the boundaries of species.

It's as if nature, in its infinite wisdom, developed this universal language of joy long before humans added words to the mix.

In our Second Prime, understanding this deeper truth about laughter adds another layer to its significance. When we laugh together, we're not just sharing a moment; we're participating in one of life's oldest and most beautiful languages, one that reminds us of our place in the great family of living beings and belonging.

When someone says "laughter is the best medicine," they're not just sharing folk wisdom. They are echoing a truth that reaches back to the foundations of medicine itself. Hippocrates, the father of modern medicine, prescribed humor therapy to his patients in 400 BCE, using jesters and musicians to lift their spirits. Ancient Greek hospitals even had dedicated spaces for comedy performances, understanding intuitively what science now confirms in fascinating detail.

Let's peek inside your body during a good laugh to see what's happening. Every chuckle is triggering two of your immune system's most powerful defenders—immunoglobulins and natural killer cells. These microscopic warriors respond to laughter like an army receiving orders. Immunoglobulins increase by 14 percent, patrolling your bloodstream and identifying potential threats. Even more impressive, your natural killer cells (think of them as your immune system's elite special forces) boost their activity by a whopping 40 percent. To put that in perspective, this is the kind of immune enhancement that pharmaceutical companies spend billions trying to achieve through medication.

That's why, when researchers at Loma Linda University discovered these numbers, it changed how we think about the relationship between joy and health. Our forebears' intuitive understanding of laughter's healing power has now been validated by modern science. When you laugh, you're not just experiencing a moment of pleasure; you're giving your immune system a power-up that keeps working long after the laughter fades.

Think of the last time you laughed so hard with a friend that your cheeks hurt. If you're a woman in your Second Prime, this possibly triggered what I like to call the giggle-piddles. Bladder control and belly laughs, it turns out, have an interesting relationship that no one warned us about. There's a world of difference between these experiences, and science is finally catching up to what our bodies have always known.

Studies reveal something remarkable about our capacity for joy and connection through shared laughter . . . even when that laughter comes with a dash of pelvic floor anxiety. It turns out our emotional intelligence—that subtle ability to read rooms, understand unspoken currents, and navigate life's complexities—gets a profound boost when we laugh together. While watching funny videos alone might give us a moment's amusement, just fifteen minutes of genuine shared laughter rewires our neural pathways more effectively than hours of solitary scrolling.

Think about those moments when humor breaks through during a difficult conversation, how a shared laugh can suddenly make space for new understanding. It's as if nature designed laughter to be both our shield and our bridge, protecting us from life's inevitable storms while creating pathways to deeper connection. The beauty of laughter in our Second Prime is that we've lived long enough to find humor in the perfectly imperfect moments: the unexpected snorts, the makeup-ruining tears of hilariousness, and even those moments when our bladders betray us. We understand that humor isn't just about being entertaining; it's about embracing our shared humanity, complete with all its messy, joyful, and occasionally damp reality.

Think of humor and laughter as emotional alchemy; the ability to transform ordinary moments into gold through the simple yet profound act of shared joy. This isn't about denying difficulty or masking pain. It's about developing the wisdom to hold both the serious and the light, knowing that often our deepest connections form in the space between the two.

When we gather with friends and the phones stay in purses and pockets, when stories flow freely and laughter bubbles up unexpectedly, we're not just passing time. We're actively engaging in one of life's most powerful forms of healing. These moments of genuine connection, of shared humor and unguarded joy, do more than just lift our spirits. They remind us that growing older doesn't mean growing serious. In fact, our Second Prime might just be when we finally perfect the art of not taking ourselves too seriously while taking life's precious moments to heart.

So, here's to the conversations that lose track of time, the laughter that makes our cheeks hurt, and the connections that remind us why we're here—to share this remarkable journey with others, finding joy in both the profound moments and the delightfully absurd ones that make life worth living.

Challenge: Explore Your World of Connections

As we close this chapter on connection, humor, and the profound impact they have on our well-being, let's pause to consider how we might bring these insights into our daily lives. The science is clear: Strong social bonds and shared laughter aren't just nice-to-haves, they're fundamental ingredients for thriving in our Second Prime. But knowing something intellectually and living it intentionally are two different journeys.

So, this week, explore your world of connections through three lenses. Remember, this isn't about perfectly executed social plans. It's about small, consistent choices that prioritize genuine connection. Start with one action that feels most natural to you. Let each authentic connection remind you that in our Second Prime, we have both the wisdom to recognize what matters and the freedom to choose it.

Belonging

- **Map Your Joy Sources:** Who makes you laugh until your cheeks hurt? Who remembers to ask about that thing you mentioned three weeks ago? These are your core connections. Nurture them intentionally.

- **Schedule One Deep Conversation:** Choose someone you've been meaning to really connect with and set aside uninterrupted time (phones away!) for a proper catch-up.

- **Create a Regular Connection Ritual:** Whether it's a weekly walk, monthly dinner club, or daily check-in with a friend, build connection into your routine.

Growth

- **Step Into Something New:** Join that class you've been eyeing or try that community group that intrigues you. New connections often bloom in unexpected places.

- **Revive a Dormant Friendship:** Think of someone who once brought joy to your life. Send that message you've been meaning to write.

- **Practice Present-Moment Connection:** During your next conversation, notice when your mind wanders to your to-do list. Gently bring your attention back to the person in front of you.

Giving

- **Be the Connection Catalyst:** Introduce two people who might enjoy knowing each other. Sometimes the greatest gift is building bridges between others.

- **Share Your Story:** When someone asks, "How are you?" resist the automatic "fine." Share something real, even if it's small. Real connection starts with real sharing.

- **Create Laughter Opportunities:** Plan activities that naturally encourage shared joy, game nights, comedy shows, or simply coffee with a friend, especially the one that is easy to laugh with.

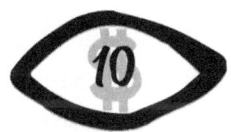

The Currency of Compound Experience: Investing in Your Second Prime

Money talks, as they say, but its voice changes as we age, maturing from the brash certainty of youth to the nuanced whispers of experience. At forty-five, it speaks of possibilities yet to unfold; at sixty, it murmurs about security while we question our place in this rapidly shifting world. Yet, in our Second Prime, we're leaning toward a changing focus—one that seeks not just accumulation but meaning.

The stakes feel deeply personal, as intimate as the questions we ask ourselves in reflective, solitary moments when we think about our purpose and what we will leave behind. Yet the ripples of our choices extend far beyond our individual shores. Each time one of us chooses to remain engaged, to start a new venture, or to challenge outdated assumptions about aging, we help chart a course for generations to follow.

Standing at this intersection of personal meaning and economic reality, we face a unique moment in history. Our generation holds unprecedented financial influence—controlling approximately 83 percent of global financial assets—yet this statistic tells only part of our story. The more compelling narrative lies in how we choose to use this influence, not just as economic actors, but as pioneers reimagining what it means to age with purpose and continued engagement.

I often think about my mother's generation, with their ceramic piggy banks and promises of predictable pension-funded futures. Their financial story followed a well-worn path with clear signposts and destinations. But our generation? We're writing a different narrative, one where the very notion of retirement has become as personal as a fingerprint, shaped by individual circumstances, dreams, and necessities.

We're living in an unprecedented moment of economic transformation. While some in our generation hold significant wealth and influence, many of us face the challenge of reinventing ourselves in a landscape where traditional retirement may be neither possible nor desirable. We're all players in a game where the rules are being rewritten as we play. Some have more pieces on the board than others, but everyone faces the same fundamental question: How do we create meaning and security in our Second Prime?

Although this story usually starts with economics, it's far more than that. It's about the unique moment we occupy in history. Whether we're financially secure or navigating uncertainty, we all face the same core questions about value, purpose, and how we choose to grow older. The workplace of tomorrow is taking shape in the choices we make today. When we remain curious and forward-thinking, sharing expertise and mentoring younger colleagues in pursuit of mutual learning, we bring our whole selves—equanimity, wisdom, and wonder—to every interaction. We help create spaces where all ages can thrive.

The data reveals that our Second Prime might be the hidden season when our creative genius reaches its most powerful expression, and our impact can have wide-reaching effects. Think of it as having played enough games to understand the deeper patterns. While younger entrepreneurs often race toward quick exits and rapid scaling, grabbing headlines and magazine covers, those of us in our Second Prime tend to build more sustainable, meaningful ventures. We're not just creating businesses; we're crafting legacies that align with our hard-won wisdom about what truly matters.

The story of aging isn't written in black and white but in subtle shades that shift dramatically when viewed through the lens of gender. Like light passing through a prism, our experience of growing older splits into distinctly different paths for women and men, each carrying its own unique challenges and unexpected gifts.

Consider this paradox: Women typically live longer—eighty-one years compared to men's seventy-six years in the U.S.—yet face steeper economic challenges in these bonus years. This reality shapes individual stories and the larger narrative of how society values and supports us as we age.

The statistics paint a portrait of persistent inequality: Women aged fifty-five and above make up 60.5 percent of new female entrants to the U.S. workforce, yet they often find themselves in positions that underutilize their expertise and undervalue their worth. The World Economic Forum's sobering projection that gender parity lies 135.6 years in the future isn't just a number—it's a call to action for our generation and those that follow.

The journey into Second Prime often brings unexpected plot twists for men. Those who've spent decades building careers in the spotlight of societal approval suddenly find themselves grappling with an unfamiliar shadow—ageism. Nearly 40 percent encounter age-related obstacles in their career advancement, a particularly bitter pill for those who've never tasted discrimination's sharp edge.

Yet within these challenges lie seeds of transformation. Women, battle-tested by years of navigating multiple biases, often demonstrate remarkable resilience in the face of age discrimination. This isn't just survival—it's hard-earned wisdom that transforms obstacles into stepping stones. The very multiplicity of roles that society expects women to juggle—caregiver, professional, family anchor—can become a source of strength, providing diverse wells of fulfillment and identity beyond the workplace.

But here's where the story takes an unexpected turn toward hope: Entrepreneurship in our Second Prime shows promising signs of leveling the playing field. Women-owned businesses boast a 69.5 percent crowdfunding success rate compared to 61.4 percent for men-owned ventures. Even more telling, women-led startups return seventy-eight cents per dollar invested, dramatically outperforming the thirty-one cents returned by male-founded companies.

Entrepreneurs over fifty consistently outperform their younger counterparts, suggesting that our Second Prime might be our most potent period for creation and contribution. Consider Arianna Huffington, who founded *The Huffington Post* at fifty-five, or Wally Blume, who launched his multimillion-dollar Denali Flavors ice cream company at fifty-seven. Ray Kroc was fifty-two when he opened his first McDonald's, and Martha Stewart was in her fifties when she built her media empire and is still going strong at eighty-three, showing us all what a Second and Third Prime look like. This isn't just about individual success stories. The Second Primer has the agency to rewrite the cultural script around aging and gender. When a woman in her sixties launches a successful venture, or a man finds a new purpose beyond traditional career definitions, they're not just changing their story but creating new possibilities for everyone who follows.

The path forward is about something other than waiting for society to change its perception of aging. It's about recognizing that our Second Prime offers unique advantages—perspective, experience, resilience—that transcend traditional barriers. Whether through entrepreneurship, mentorship, or innovative new career paths, we have the opportunity to create economic models that honor the full spectrum of human potential, regardless of age or gender.

I've come to understand that our Second Prime journey

is about something other than the size of our bank accounts or investment portfolios. It's about reimagining our relationship with everything we value—purpose, contribution, connection—at precisely the moment when we have the wisdom to understand what truly matters. Whether we're retiring comfortably or reinventing ourselves out of necessity, we're all part of a generation that's redefining what it means to age with purpose and dignity.

The road in front of us isn't marked by the traditional milestones our parents followed. Instead, we're creating new ways of remaining vital and engaged, adapting to challenges that previous generations never faced. This is where our story becomes not just interesting, but essential. We're pioneering approaches to longevity and purpose that will shape the journey for generations to come.

Our Second Prime isn't merely about managing what we've accumulated—it's about reimagining what becomes possible when wisdom meets opportunity, when experience finds new purpose, and when we fully embrace our power to shape tomorrow's story.

Looking ahead to 2050, demographers project that over two billion people worldwide will be sixty or older—a number that promises significant global challenges. Imagine standing in a room where one in every four people embodies the wisdom of their Second Prime. This isn't just a statistical shift; it's a fundamental reimagining of what it means to be part of society. The traditional notion of retirement—that gentle fading into the background our parents were promised—feels like an ill-fitting garment from another era.

This demographic transformation requires us to be actively engaged—simply adapting with a go-along mentality is not sustainable. This seismic shift in demographics does more than beckon; it insists on innovation, creating new pathways for contribution that honor our accumulated wisdom and our hunger for continued growth.

Yet, here's where the story takes an interesting turn. While businesses increasingly struggle to find talent, many still hold fast to outdated biases about age and capability. The most forward-thinking companies are beginning to recognize what we've known all along—that diverse teams spanning generations, genders, and experiences bring a richness of perspective that no homogeneous group can match.

I've witnessed this transformation firsthand in workplaces where wisdom and fresh perspective meld together, where the energy of youth combines with the steady hand of experience to create something extraordinary. These aren't just feel-good stories; they're blueprints for the future of work itself.

The path forward is more than just demanding space at tables designed for younger generations. It's about building new tables altogether, ones that celebrate the unique alchemy that happens when different life stages converge. Whether in traditional employment, entrepreneurship, or completely new models of con-tribution we haven't yet imagined, our role is to be architects of change rather than passive observers.

This is where our inconvenient dreams come into play. Those persistent whispers of possibility that won't let us settle for less than full engagement with life, regardless of our age or circum-stance. Every time one of us chooses to learn a new skill, start a venture, or step into a role that challenges age-based expectations, we help rewrite the story of what's possible in our Second Prime.

What if, at eighteen, you knew that sixty wasn't an ending but a deliberate beginning? Picture this truth: Your early career is simply the first act, gathering momentum for a second, third, or fourth renaissance when you'll learn what truly calls to you. This isn't about retiring from life but about stepping fully into it, filled with self-love, experience, and wisdom, ready to pursue what has always whispered in your quietest moments.

How would this change everything? It fosters a life lived not in a straight line toward retirement but in an expansive spiral upward where experience and wonder meet, where your Second Prime becomes not a finish line but a threshold to cross with purpose and anticipation of the gifts that have been dormant within you.

This evolution isn't just about fighting for our place in traditional structures. It's about recognizing that some of the most profound contributions come through unexpected channels. It could be the former executive who now teaches conflict resolution in community centers, or the retired engineer who mentors social entrepreneurs. It could be the parent returning to the workforce, bringing decades of life management skills to a new profession.

The path forward requires both courage and creativity. It asks us to question deeply held assumptions—not just society's but our own. When we catch ourselves thinking, *I'm too old to start something new*, or *that's a young person's game*, we're reading from an outdated script. The new story we're writing together recognizes that innovation doesn't belong to any age. It belongs to those brave enough to remain curious, engaged, and slightly uncomfortable with the status quo.

Education takes on new meaning in this context. Learning becomes not just a means to an end but also a declaration of continued engagement with life's possibilities. Every new skill mastered, every fresh perspective gained, becomes another tool for our reinvention. The workplace evolution we're witnessing isn't just about policies or procedures. It's about reimagining the essence of contribution. Each time a company welcomes the perspective of a Second Prime employee, each time a team benefits from cross-generational collaboration, we move closer to a world where wisdom and innovation dance together in perfect rhythm.

Think of our generation as bridge builders. We stand at a unique moment in history, able to translate between the traditions we inherited and the future taking shape before us. Our most significant contribution might not be in what we know but in how we help different generations, perspectives, and approaches find common ground.

Does the relationship with technological revolutions feel like it's leaving us behind? It's offering us unprecedented opportunities to share our wisdom in new ways. A lifetime of experience can now reach around the globe through digital platforms, touching lives and solving problems we never imagined we could reach. Yet we understand something crucial that younger generations are still discovering; technology is a tool, not a replacement for human connection and wisdom.

We are not digital natives but mindful immigrants to this new landscape—carriers of a disappearing memory. We remember afternoons that stretched uninterrupted by notifications, conversations that unfolded without the subtle anxiety of devices waiting to be checked. This isn't mere nostalgia but a vital remembrance of human rhythms that align with our deeper nature.

This intersection of seasoned perspective and digital reach deserves a deeper exploration than these pages can contain, but its significance cannot be overlooked. We stand at a unique crossroads where our accumulated wisdom meets unprecedented connectivity. The Second Prime generation remembers a world before screens mediated our existence—we've witnessed the birth of the digital age with eyes already accustomed to recognizing patterns across decades, not just trending algorithms. This gives us a distinctive vantage point from which we can harness these tools without being defined by them.

As the analog natives dwindle—those who knew a world before the constant digital hum—we carry something precious: the knowledge of how thought deepens in sustained silence, how presence feels when undivided by screens. Perhaps in our Second

Prime, we're uniquely positioned to create these oases of undistracted attention, not by rejecting technology but by remembering its proper place in a well-lived life.

We might find ourselves becoming unexpected guardians of something essential: teaching by example how to set deliberate boundaries around our digital engagement. Not to turn away from progress but to preserve the spaces where human wisdom has always flourished: in the pause, the silence, the unmediated moment of genuine connection.

As the tools become more advanced, our relationship with work itself is being redefined. No longer bound by traditional career trajectories, we're free to explore purpose-driven engagement, finding ways to contribute that align with our deepest values and highest aspirations. Whether that means starting a business that solves a problem we've observed, mentoring the next generation, or pioneering novel approaches to old challenges, the key is remaining actively engaged with life's possibilities.

The barriers we face—ageism, outdated assumptions, systemic biases—are real. But they're not immovable. This is more than a chapter in a book; it's a gentle provocation asking you to unravel everything you've assumed about the relationship between calendar pages and human vitality. Consider this your permission slip to reimagine what work means when untethered from conventional timelines, to rediscover purpose beyond traditional career narratives, and to recognize that your contributions haven't reached their expiration date—you've barely begun your most interesting chapter. Above all, this is your invitation to a gathering already in progress: a collective reimagining of what it means to grow older with fierce grace, renewed clarity, and a voice that's only grown more resonant with the passage of time.

Your inconvenient dream—that persistent *tap-tap-tap* of possibility that won't let you rest—isn't a distraction from your proper path. It is your path, illuminated by decades of experience and ready to guide you toward your next great adventure. The world desperately needs the unique combination of wisdom and possibility that only Second Primers can offer.

Consider the difference between mindlessly consuming content versus thoughtfully crafting resources that address real needs in your field of expertise. When you share hard-won insights from decades of experience, detailed how-to guides that help others master complex skills, or thoughtful analysis of industry trends, you're not just adding to the noise. You're creating lasting value. This isn't about chasing likes or followers but extending your natural role as a mentor and guide into the digital realm, where your knowledge can reach those who need it most.

We have a unique opportunity to significantly impact society and establish our relevance and value by continuing to serve throughout our entire lifespan. Use your knowledge and expertise to drive innovation and progress; there are unmet needs in society that you can fulfill. What gifts and skills are calling you to action? If not now, when will you pursue your inconvenient dreams or explore new opportunities without hesitation? Take some time in contemplation and reflection to look at the big picture. Second Primers must stay economically engaged for Social Security's solvency. How will you contribute to this societal need for economic participation?

Your inconvenient dream is your guide and can soon become your calling. The call will get louder and louder the closer you get to the spark that ignites your desired future. It is important to note that your dream is a valuable antidote to many of life's challenges, and it keeps the pre-programmed negative feelings about aging from taking root in your garden.

Every successful venture launched by someone over fifty sends ripples through our cultural narrative about aging, challenging assumptions, and opening doors for others to follow. But let's be clear: This isn't about starting businesses merely for profit. It's about recognizing that our accumulated wisdom, battle scars, and deeply personal understanding of human needs create a unique formula for success. When we align our ventures with our inconvenient dreams, we tap into something more powerful than market opportunity.

The Ewing Marion Kauffman Foundation's research is more than just reporting statistics when it shows increasing entrepreneurship among those ages fifty-five to sixty-four. It's documenting a quiet revolution where life experience gets the recognition it deserves as a crucial ingredient for success.

As we stand at this intersection of experience and opportunity, the question isn't whether you should pursue an entrepreneurial path but how you will use our unique advantages to create a Second Prime that you desire. The point made by the data is not to assume everyone wants to start a business; rather, it is to make clear that you have limitless capabilities in your Second Prime. The world needs the unique blend of knowledge, expertise, and innovation that only you can offer—solutions shaped by decades of real-world understanding and tempered by the insight that true success transcends mere financial metrics.

There's a profound liberation in realizing that our "too late" years are precisely the right time. Our relationship with work in Second Prime demands more than just adaptation—it calls for reinvention. The traditional chronological resume with its linear storytelling often fails to capture the rich complexity of our accumulated wisdom. What's needed is a new way to articulate our value, one that honors both our experience and our potential.

Enter the *Wisdom Profile*—a powerful reframing of how we present ourselves to the world. Where traditional resumes list positions held, this approach weaves together the profound insights gained from decades of lived experience with our capacity for continued growth. Most importantly, it demonstrates something uniquely valuable: pattern recognition refined by years of engagement. Where others might see isolated incidents, we perceive interconnected systems. Where they spot immediate problems, we recognize underlying opportunities.

Consider how our relationship with risk has evolved through these years. While society might assume we become more conservative with age, many of us discover an unexpected boldness. The data confirms what our instincts suggest—our ventures tend to survive longer and create more sustainable value precisely because of this seasoned perspective.

Across kitchens and home offices, Second Primers are creating new models of contribution. A former executive discovers her calling in teaching mindfulness to burned-out professionals. A retired engineer finds unexpected joy in creating artisanal furniture. These aren't mere career changes. They're expressions of authenticity that have waited for their moment.

The elephant in the employment room remains a pervasive ageist attitude about hiring and retaining older employees. Yet transformation rarely announces itself with fanfare. Instead, it speaks through quiet moments when we dare to question what we've always assumed about aging, purpose, and contribution. The path ahead isn't a single highway but a web of trails, each one blazed by those who refused to accept the traditional story of decline.

Some changes feel beyond our grasp, like shifting societal norms, reimagining retirement, rebuilding institutions. Yet within these sweeping transformations lies an intimate truth—we each hold the power to rewrite our own story. Whether from a boardroom or a kitchen table, we're all architects of what comes next, drawing blueprints with the ink of experience.

The future beckons not with certainty but with possibility. It invites us to:

- reimagine retirement as a fluid transition rather than a final destination;
- challenge the stubborn roots of ageist thinking in our workplaces;
- advocate for policies that recognize the value of seasoned contributors; and
- most importantly, pursue our inconvenient dreams, those persistent visions of purpose that refuse to fade with time.

Challenge: Explore the Wisdom Profile

To translate this philosophy into practical action, let's explore the essential components that make a Wisdom Profile incredibly powerful:

1. **Executive Summary of Impact:** Begin with a powerful narrative that weaves together your most significant achievements and the wisdom they've generated. Rather than listing jobs, tell the story of problems you've solved and the insights you've gained.

2. **Core Competencies Section:** Create categories that highlight transferable skills:
   - Leadership wisdom (team building, conflict resolution, strategic planning)
   - Technical mastery (specific skills relevant to your target role)
   - Cross-cultural understanding (global experience, working across generations)

○ Crisis management (times you've navigated significant challenges)

3. **Life Experience Portfolio:** Instead of a traditional work history, create impact stories that demonstrate your value:

   ○ Major projects and outcomes

   ○ Innovation initiatives

   ○ Mentorship success stories

   ○ Community leadership roles

   ○ Personal growth milestones

4. **Continuous Learning Journey:** Highlight recent training, certifications, or self-directed learning to demonstrate your commitment to growth and adaptation.

5. **Wisdom in Action:** Include specific examples of how your experience has directly contributed to:

   ○ Cost savings

   ○ Process improvements

   ○ Team development and leadership

   ○ Problem-solving

   ○ Innovation

WISDOM PROFILE EXAMPLE
Mathematician, Life Architect, and Growth Catalyst

Executive Summary of Impact

Through twenty-five years of weaving together classroom dynamics, family orchestration, and community care, I've developed a unique talent for transforming complex systems into elegant solutions. My journey has taught me that the most profound insights often emerge from the intersection of seemingly unrelated domains, whether solving algebraic equations, optimizing a family budget, or reimagining support systems for cancer patients.

Core Competencies & Patterns of Insight

Resource Optimization & Financial Stewardship

- Developed innovative budget-stretching strategies that enabled enriching family experiences while managing education costs for three children
- Created and implemented efficient household management systems that seamlessly integrate elder care responsibilities with professional commitments
- Designed a departmental resource allocation system that reduced textbook costs by 30 percent while improving student access to materials

Human-Centered Problem Solving

- Cultivated an ability to translate abstract mathematical concepts into relatable real-world applications, improving student engagement and comprehension
- Pioneered a peer support network within the cancer charity that increased volunteer retention by 40 percent
- Developed flexible caregiving schedules that honor both elder parents' dignity and family members' needs

Systems Design & Implementation

- Transformed garden planning into a mathematical model for sustainable yield and resource management
- Created modular lesson plans that adapt to diverse learning styles while maintaining curriculum integrity

- Designed volunteer coordination systems that maximize impact while respecting contributors' time constraints

Expertise in Action: Key Achievements

Education & Mentorship

- Guided over two thousand students through mathematical discovery, with 85 percent reporting increased confidence in problem-solving abilities
- Mentored twelve new teachers in classroom management and curriculum development
- Created differentiated learning approaches that improved test scores by 25 percent among struggling students

Community Impact & Leadership

- Developed and implemented a mentor-matching program for the cancer support network
- Transformed the school's math club into a community service initiative, where students apply mathematical concepts to local challenges
- Successfully balanced multiple life roles while maintaining professional excellence and personal growth

Continuous Learning Journey

- Currently exploring permaculture design principles to integrate mathematical modeling with sustainable gardening
- Developing a workshop series called Life Mathematics: Applied Problem-Solving for Real-World Challenges
- Studying innovative approaches to elder care and intergenerational living

Available for consultation on: Educational Program Design | Resource Optimization | Community Program Development | Systems Integration | Life-Work Balance Strategies

Remember, your Wisdom Profile should confidently highlight the unique perspective and capabilities that only decades of experience can provide. Focus on how your accumulated wisdom makes you uniquely qualified to oversee complex challenges and guide others toward success.

As we stand at this intersection of wisdom and possibility, our paths forward take different forms. Some of us hold the power to reshape organizational cultures directly, while others craft more personal revolutions. Yet each path shares the same profound truth—our Second Prime isn't about fitting into existing structures, but about reimagining what's possible when experience meets opportunity. Here are some examples to get you reimagining.

For Those Shaping Organizations: Architects of Change

If you sit in boardrooms, lead teams, or influence organizational decisions, you hold unique power to reshape how society values wisdom. Your position offers opportunities to create ripples that extend far beyond individual careers:

- **Implement Inclusive Hiring Practices:** Imagine workplaces not as rigid structures, but as living, breathing organisms capable of perpetual reinvention. The most profound transformations begin with a fundamental shift in perception—seeing age not as a limitation, but as a reservoir of accumulated wisdom. Recognize the value of experience and the unique perspectives that older workers can bring to the team.

- **Facilitate Job Redesign:** Whether you are a business owner or an employee seeking to adapt roles or create new positions that cater to the strengths and abilities of older workers, consider the subtle art of job redesign as a form of collective imagination. It's about seeing roles not as fixed containers but as fluid opportunities for human capability. An experienced professional isn't simply seeking accommodation—they're offering a lifetime of nuanced understanding.

- **Promote Workplace Flexibility:** Offer part-time, remote, or flexible working arrangements. This can help older workers balance their work with other aspects of life, such as health issues or caregiving responsibilities.

- **Encourage Lifelong Learning and Career Development:** Invest in continuous training and education to keep older workers up to date with industry trends and technologies. This can help them stay competitive and relevant in the job market.

- **Promote a Mentoring Culture:** Leverage the experience and knowledge of older workers by encouraging them to mentor younger employees. This can facilitate knowledge transfer and foster a culture of mutual respect and learning.

For Those Charting Personal Transformations: Pioneers of Purpose

Perhaps your revolution begins at your kitchen table, in quiet moments of contemplation about what comes next. Your journey may feel more personal, but it's no less powerful in reshaping our cultural narrative about aging and work.

- **Embrace Your Wisdom Profile:** Traditional chronological resumes often don't serve Second Primers well, as they can inadvertently highlight age rather than expertise. Invest time in creating your Wisdom Profile. This is a strategic presentation of your accumulated knowledge, skills, and life experiences that positions you as a valuable asset to any organization.

- **Consider Unconventional Paths:** The traditional notion of retirement—that gentle fading into the background our parents were promised—feels like something from another time. Instead, explore what happens when you align your accumulated wisdom with society's unmet needs.

- **Leverage Digital Platforms:** In our digital age, technology offers powerful tools for sharing your wisdom and creating meaningful impact. Consider approaching digital spaces not as entertainment venues but as lecture halls, mentorship spaces, and communities of practice where your accumulated wisdom can truly serve others.

- **Build Cross-Generational Bridges:** Foster intergenerational collaboration and knowledge sharing. Your ability to translate between traditions and emerging trends makes you an invaluable bridge builder in our rapidly changing world.

Together, these paths—whether organizational or personal—create a journey of transformation that extends far beyond individual careers. They represent our collective opportunity to reshape not just how society views aging but how we harness the profound potential of human wisdom across all life stages.

Challenge: What Gifts Do I Bring?

Revisit your inconvenient dream and imagine how you might incorporate the following suggestions to bring your gifts to the world:

- How can sharing your expertise by becoming a mentor or consultant in your field enrich your professional life and that of others?

- How can you utilize digital media to disseminate your knowledge and skills to a broader audience?

- How can you redefine retirement as a transformative period, potentially leading to starting your own business?

- What measures can you take to advocate for age diversity and inclusivity in the workplace, and why is this important?

- How can your perspective or knowledge fulfill an unmet need?

- What are some nontraditional career paths that require the human touch, and how do they align with your skills and experience?

- How can engaging in community service or joining a board or committee drive change within your field of expertise or community?

- What might pursuing a second career as a teacher, mentor, or educator in your area of expertise look like, and how could this benefit you and others?

- How can you challenge stereotypes about aging and lead by example in your professional and personal lives?

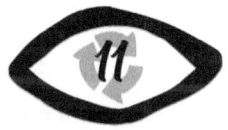

From Target Market to Market Maker: Flipping the Script on Aging Narratives

Stories shape our world in ways we rarely pause to consider while absorbing them. They whisper to us through billboard advertisements, echo in our social media feeds, and dance across our screens big and small. Each one leaves an invisible yet undeniable imprint on how we see others, ourselves, and our place in the world. I've been thinking lately about the stories we're told about aging and, more importantly, the stories we agree to and unknowingly incorporate into our world view.

The other day, I found myself lingering in front of my magnified mirror, examining the subtle lines that mark my journey through time, noticing how my face was not what it once was, heavier on one side and saggy in the jawline. What's not so subtle is the endless inner voice identifying areas to improve—a brown spot here, a slight droop there. Should I have a lower facelift? The silent dialogue is relentless, a constant negotiation between acceptance and resistance. I yearn to not give a damn! I am actively seeking balance, self-love, self-care, and self-acceptance as I grow older. But maintaining equilibrium is an unending battle when the marketing machine has other plans.

In that intimate moment of self-reflection, something shifted. Like catching a glimpse of the puppet master's strings, I suddenly saw how deeply marketing narratives had choreographed this daily ritual of self-scrutiny. How many times had I heard that the lines on my face needed to be fought, reversed, or eliminated? The language reveals a deeper story that positions aging as an enemy to be vanquished rather than a journey to be embraced.

This revelation led me to the illuminating work of marketing sage Seth Godin, whose insights about human behavior cast a new light on my mirror moment. He speaks about how we're fundamentally wired for status seeking and tribal belonging, our brains constantly scanning our environment for cues about where we fit or don't fit in the social hierarchy. Through this lens, my morning mirror ritual transformed from a simple grooming routine into something more profound: a daily engagement with internalized stories about status, belonging, and worth.

We are, at our core, storytelling creatures seeking belonging. The narratives we absorb shape not just how we see ourselves but how we move through the world. For too long, the story of aging has been one of declining status, a narrative that whispers *less than instead of equal to*, that frames each passing year as a step down rather than a step forward in life's journey.

I remember the first time I truly understood how deeply status seeking was woven into the fabric of my choices: the entertainment I seek, the countless items I buy (shoes, bags, skincare, makeup, and more), and the place where I live. This invisible influence is a powerful force that permeates every part of our lives.

As Godin illustrates, every purchase we make, every brand we align with, and every social media post we like becomes part of an intricate language of social positioning. Choosing to opt out is also a social positioning action. These aren't shallow choices; they're expressions of our deeply human need to find our place in the world.

If we are attuned, if we truly recognize *why* we do *what* we do, we can find profound clarity that transforms how we see ourselves and the world around us. For me, that clarity arrived with understanding Godin's work and questioning some of my consumer choices. I looked around at my favorite things: a beloved scarf, a handbag, face cream at my bedside. Each item represented not just a purchase but a desire to be in the know, have a connection, and be seen.

The revelation was both liberating and profound. Like discovering a new language, I began to see how each purchase becomes part of the story we're telling about who we are, what matters to us, and how we want to be seen. It's not about judgment or shame. It's about understanding the beautiful complexity of human nature and our intense and innate desire to belong.

What's fascinating is how this understanding intersects with our journey into Second Prime. Society has traditionally drafted a limited story about aging that equates advancing years with declining relevance. We've all felt its subtle influence in the marketing messages that promise to help us stay young, in the pressure to appear ageless, in the constant push to prove we're still in the game.

But here's where our Second Prime wisdom becomes transformative. Understanding the status dynamics doesn't mean we need to reject them. Instead, it empowers us to consciously, thoughtfully choose which stories we want to be part of. In fact, seeing the status game for what it is and deciding how we want to play it is part of the joy of growing older. This is the joy of wisdom that comes with age. We can brim with confidence, aware of the powerful undercurrent that shapes our behaviors. It's a deep source of confidence and comfort. We can appreciate beautiful things while knowing their true value lies not in the status they confer but in the enjoyment they bring us. At the same time, we can expand beyond the traditional status-seeking behavior and choose to belong to groups that celebrate growth, wisdom, and authenticity rather than chasing an endless loop of youth-focused games.

This awareness opens exciting possibilities. What if we redefined status around the qualities that naturally increase with age: wisdom, experience, perspective, and the ability to model behavior that signals evolution and growth? What if we created new groups centered not on external markers but on internal growth, contribution, and the courage to pursue our inconvenient dreams?

The data reveals a powerful shift in how age-positive messaging resonates in the marketplace. Nielsen's research shows that brands celebrating authentic aging and meaningful contributions by older adults see their engagement rates rise by 157 percent compared to traditional advertising approaches. This impact goes beyond mere representation. Meta's business insights reveal that age-positive content receives 2.3 times more meaningful interactions and shares. When brands feature genuine, non-stereotypical portrayals of people over fifty, research shows an 85 percent increase in positive brand perception.

These striking metrics aren't just numbers; they reflect a fundamental transformation where older adults are no longer passive consumers but active architects of a new aging narrative in the modern world.

This shift isn't just about personal vanity or social positioning. It has profound implications for how we see ourselves and navigate our Second Prime. When we free ourselves from outdated status games, we create space for more authentic forms of connection and contribution. We stop asking, *Do I still matter?* and start declaring, *This is how I choose to matter.*

The research backs this up. Brands that position aging as a journey of increasing rather than decreasing status see customer loyalty increase by 48 percent. They're tapping into a profound truth—that our hunger for status and belonging can be satisfied not by chasing youth but by embracing the unique power of our accumulated wisdom. The data tells its own compelling story. While those of us in our Second Prime control a fifteen-trillion-dollar market, traditional marketing narratives have often relegated us to the margins. It's a fascinating disconnect. We hold immense economic power, yet traditionally, the stories being told about us usually feel as if they are written from a distance, through a lens of diminishment rather than celebration.

The narratives we consume shape more than our buying habits; they influence our very sense of possibility. When we see vibrant, engaged individuals in their Second Prime leading adventures, starting businesses, falling in love, starting late-in-life families, or reinventing themselves, these stories become permission slips for our transformation.

Research from behavioral psychology shows that we make decisions based on the stories we believe about ourselves and our place in the world. Consider Diana Nyad, who at age sixty-four became the first person to swim from Cuba to Florida without a shark cage, completing the 110-mile journey that had eluded her in her younger years. But the real impact wasn't just in her achievement; it was in how her story transformed the narratives of countless other adults in their Second Prime. Following her historic swim, swimming clubs across the country reported a surge in enrollment among people over fifty, many explicitly citing Nyad's example as their inspiration.

These individuals weren't just joining in to swim; they were rewriting their own stories from *I'm too old to start something new* to *I'm just getting started.* The ripple effect continued as these new swimmers shared their experiences on social media and within their communities, creating a self-reinforcing cycle of positive aging narratives. When marketing consistently presents aging as a journey of decline, it creates a self-fulfilling prophecy. But when we see ourselves reflected in stories of growth, wisdom, and continued evolution, our behaviors naturally align with these more empowering narratives.

Each campaign that celebrates the fullness of aging helps dismantle the invisible barriers we've internalized, transforming *I could never* into *Why not me?* Carefully crafted photographs or cleverly written taglines can be more than marketing campaigns for products. They can be bridges between our present selves and our Second Prime potential. With its staggering 58.5-billion-dollar valuation, the global anti-aging industry speaks volumes about our collective relationship with youth, beauty, and time. Like a mirror that shows only shadows, it has reduced the richness of human evolution into a series of problems awaiting their bottled solutions. Yet within this narrowed narrative lies a profound invitation to rebellion, to authorship, to transformation.

Consider how marketing, when wielded with wisdom and intention, has the power to be not merely a messenger but a maker of possibility. Its genuine opportunity lies not in the products it presents, but in the future it dares us to become. When we encounter images that reflect back to us not our fears but our potential, something extraordinary awakens. These glimpses of vital, engaged Second Primers living fully become more than aspirational moments. They are seeds of permission planted in the fertile soil of our collective imagination. Each authentic representation, each story of renewal and purpose, grows into a new narrative strand in the emerging story of what aging can be.

In this way, we stand at a crucial intersection between the old story of aging as a decline and the new story waiting to be told; one where our evolution isn't a problem to be solved but an adventure to be lived. The choice before us isn't just about which products to buy or which lifestyle to adopt. It's about which future we dare to nurture into being.

Marketing isn't simply a passive mirror reflecting our collective narrative. It's a force we must actively engage with and reshape. Each time we share our stories of transformation and celebrate our continued growth, we crack the foundation of outdated narratives. Our authentic voices, carrying both the weight of lived experience and the lightness of newfound freedom, can reshape cultural consciousness. Every choice we make, every story we share, ripples outward to become part of a larger narrative about aging in our modern world. We're not just characters in this unfolding story. We're its authors, its protagonists, and its living proof.

There's a delicious irony in how marketing tries to speak to us sometimes. Remember our conversations about maintaining a sense of humor through life's transitions? The same principle applies here. Some of the most successful campaigns targeting our demographic have embraced wit and wisdom over worry and fear. Brands that can laugh with us (not at us) about the journey of aging see customer loyalty increase by 62 percent. Dove's "Pro Age" campaign marked a revolutionary shift in beauty marketing. Rather than whispering about anti-aging, they boldly proclaimed, "Beauty Has No Age Limit." The campaign featured unretouched photographs of women in their fifties and sixties celebrating their bodies with confidence and joy. One striking image showed a silver-haired model laughing, accompanied by the tagline "Too old to be in an anti-aging ad"—a brilliant subversion of traditional beauty marketing that resonated deeply with consumers.

Allstate Insurance created waves with their "Experience More" campaign featuring Dennis Haysbert as a voice of authority and someone actively engaged in life's adventures. The ads playfully challenged the notion that wisdom means slowing down, showing instead how experience enhances our capacity for joy and discovery.

Some of the most potent examples come from athletic brands. Nike's "Unlimited Youth" campaign featured Sister Madonna

Buder, the "Iron Nun," who began running at age forty-eight and competed in her first IRONMAN at fifty-five. By eighty-six, she had completed forty-five IRONMANs. The campaign's genius lay in its blend of inspiration and irreverence, with Sister Buder joking about how God might be her personal trainer.

L'Oréal Paris has long championed age positivity with their "Age Perfect" ambassadors like Helen Mirren and Jane Fonda. But their "Golden Warriors" campaign truly captured the zeitgeist, featuring women over fifty speaking candidly about embracing their age while pursuing new passions. Mirren's quip, "I'm not aging; I'm maturing like a fine wine," became a viral sensation.

These campaigns succeeded because they didn't just sell products. They reflected our wisdom, vitality, and delicious defiance of outdated age narratives. They showed us not who we should be but how we are already magnificent because of our complexity, experience, and ever-evolving journey.

Our earlier discussions about contribution take on new meaning in the context of marketing and media representation. The stories being told about us shouldn't just focus on what we consume but on what we create and contribute. Yet traditional marketing often misses this crucial aspect of our identity. They see us as consumers when we're creators; as audiences when we're the agents of change. The data supports this disconnect: 82 percent of those in their Second Prime report feeling they have valuable wisdom to share, and only 24 percent of marketing content targeting this demographic acknowledges this desire to contribute.

The stories we're writing with our lives are fundamentally reshaping how marketing sees us. We're not interested in quietly fading into demographic obscurity. We're launching businesses, learning new skills, engaging in our community, and reimagining what's possible. Consider the link between marketing and modern entrepreneurship—the Second Prime generation is rewriting what's possible. The Kauffman Foundation tells us a remarkable story: Individuals aged fifty-five to sixty-four have consistently led entrepreneurial activity in America for the past decade. But numbers, while powerful, only sketch the outline of a deeper truth we're witnessing unfold in our own circles and lives.

Sarah, at fifty-eight, transformed her environmental consulting experience into a thriving sustainability start-up. Jason's retirement from education became the launchpad for an EdTech venture that's reshaping how we think about lifelong learning. These aren't outliers; they're mirrors reflecting our own possibilities. The Global Entrepreneurship Monitor confirms what we're seeing. Senior entrepreneurship is rising steadily worldwide, creating a visible new normal that reshapes market demographics and our collective imagination. Each visible success becomes a beacon, illuminating the path for others still harboring inconvenient dreams in the quiet corners of their hearts.

Marketing isn't just witnessing this shift—it's both shaped by it and actively shaping it in return. As the demand for more relatable voices grows, so does the need for authentic and inclusive marketing strategies.

As we've explored throughout this book, our Second Prime isn't about receding; it's about living powerfully. The media is beginning to recognize what we ourselves are deciding—that this chapter of life isn't an epilogue but a new beginning. The stories being told about us are changing because we're changing them, one authentic share, one bold choice, one inconvenient dream at a time.

Challenge: Marketing and Media Hygiene

Remember: The most powerful marketing campaign isn't found on billboards or screens. It unfolds in the daily stories we choose to live. Each time we step fully into our vitality, refusing to dim our light or shrink our dreams, we become living testaments to what's possible in our Second Prime. Your life isn't just part of this unfolding narrative. It's a beacon lighting the way for others. What story will you choose to tell today? Better yet, what story will you choose to live?

The following list offers a few ways to consider how your consumption of marketing and media might use a refresh.

- Be mindful each day. Take notice of how aging appears in the marketing messages surrounding you. Observe not just the obvious advertisements, but the subtle whispers that shape your self-perception.

- Listen carefully to the voice that speaks when you catch your reflection. Is it yours or just marketing implanting an entire vocabulary of lack that sounds eerily like your own thoughts?

- Reflect on your recent purchases and decisions. Were they born from authentic desire or based on status and belonging?

- Choose one aspect of your life where marketing has influenced your self-perception (perhaps your appearance, aging process, fitness level, or consumption habits) and actively rewrite the script to a more positive, self-affirming identity.

- Journal. Write your own authentic narrative that reclaims this territory—not as a battlefield where you've been found wanting, but as a landscape you've earned the right to define. Draft the uncensored truth of your relationship with this aspect, beyond the convenient fictions of commerce.

- Share this story in whatever way feels natural, through conversations, social media, or within your community.

Once you've started taking note of what you consume, you can start shifting it. Begin curating your media consumption to include voices that celebrate Second Prime living. As you reshape your digital landscape, seek out those who illuminate the path ahead with wisdom, humor, and authenticity. Here are some vibrant voices leading the conversation:

- Julia Louis-Dreyfus's *Wiser Than Me* podcast emerges as a masterclass in the art of deep listening and joyful curiosity. Through conversations with luminaries like Jane Fonda, Carol Burnett, and Isabel Allende, she weaves together lessons and acquired wisdom while challenging our culture's narrow definitions of aging. Each episode feels less like an interview and more like eavesdropping on an intimate conversation between friends where laughter and profound insights dance together perfectly.

- My own offering, the *Your Second Prime* podcast adds another inspirational voice to this narrative, exploring the territory where science, philosophy, and common sense meets up with lived experience. Through conversations with researchers, thought leaders, and everyday revolutionaries, it illuminates the path for those ready to embrace their most vital decades. The show doesn't just talk about transformation; it creates a space where transformation feels possible and inevitable.

- Other powerful voices include Dian Griesel, whose Silver Disobedience platform has grown from a personal blog into a movement celebrating age-positive living. Her daily reflections reach millions, offering permission to reimagine what's possible beyond fifty. Maria Shriver's Sunday Paper newsletter and her Radically Reframing Aging series provide deeply researched insights alongside personal revelations about navigating this rich territory.

- Padma Lakshmi's various platforms consistently celebrate the wisdom that comes with age, while Ming-Na Wen's social media presence joyfully demolishes stereotypes about vitality and visibility. Stanley Tucci's exploration of food, culture, and connection through his shows and books offers a masterclass in how passion knows no age limit.

- If you can't find exactly what you're looking for, become the representation you wish to see by sharing your own stories of growth and transformation.

Beyond X and Y: Reimagining Biological Differences in Our Second Prime

Captain obvious here: Aging isn't a one-size-fits-all journey. This became clear during a conversation with my friend Michael, a colleague who had always prided himself on his reserved demeanor.

"I never imagined I'd need to learn a new emotional language at sixty," he confessed. "With my parents growing older, navigating tough conversations and complex decisions with my siblings has become challenging. I'm unsure how to keep my balance." Michael described how his traditional approach to emotional situations—pushing through, staying strong, keeping quiet, ignoring feelings—had begun to exact an unexpected toll on his health and relationships. "What I'm figuring out, something I wished I had known much earlier," he added with a half-laugh, "is that the vulnerability I've been dodging might actually be . . . useful. Turns out that being able to talk about feelings and connect are tools I've ignored. And man, could I use that tool right about now."

His story reflects a truth I've encountered repeatedly in my research and personal experience. The path through our Second Prime is profoundly influenced by our sex, but not in the ways most of us expect. Scientific rescarch published in *Psychology and Aging* and longitudinal studies from the University of California reveal fascinating patterns in how male brains evolve with age. Studies show increased activation in emotion-processing regions of the brain in older men, particularly in the anterior cingulate cortex. This biological shift, combined with naturally declining testosterone levels, often leads to greater emotional awareness and expression in men during their later years. Women, by contrast, have typically developed these emotional capacities earlier through social expectations and cultural patterns. While these are general trends and individual experiences vary widely, understanding these gender-influenced paths isn't about accepting limitations. It's about understanding ourselves and claiming the power to author our own story of aging with greater wisdom and intention.

It will likely not surprise you that women outlive men in every country on Earth, with an average gap of 5.4 years. But here's what fascinates me: This isn't just about chromosomes and hormones. Our choices, the stereotypes we agree to, and the personal narratives we create about how we connect and care for ourselves profoundly shape how we age.

Think of your body as a complex instrument fine-tuned by generations of genetic wisdom. This instrument comes with built-in backup systems for women, two X chromosomes working in tandem, offering resilience that manifests in fascinating ways. Within our bodies lies an extraordinary story of stability, particularly in the feminine form. Women's immune systems show remarkable resistance to age's persistent touch, while our telomeres (those tiny guardians of cellular youth) hold their ground with quiet determination. This isn't merely touting resilience based on experiences; it's also written in our cells.

The evidence speaks through careful scientific observation. Women's immune warriors—particularly our T lymphocytes—maintain their vigilant watch well into our seventies. Our telomeres stretch longer than men's by approximately 240 base pairs, a microscopic difference that has profound implications for our journey through time. This biological advantage manifests in tangible ways, as women in their sixties and seventies have fewer hospitalizations during challenging seasons like flu outbreaks. Understanding this goes beyond simple statistics or complex cellular mechanics. We need to delve into the deeper currents of how we age and recognize that these biological gifts aren't guarantees but opportunities to shape our later years with greater awareness and intention.

For men, genetic composition tells an equally compelling story that speaks of adaptation and resilience in its own distinct voice. While the XY chromosomal pattern offers less genetic redundancy than the female counterpart, it brings unique strengths that reveal themselves particularly in the Second Prime and beyond. Scientific research shows that men's immune systems—though generally more vulnerable to seasonal ailments—demonstrate a remarkable capacity for managing inflammatory responses, a crucial factor in healthy aging. This biological pattern manifests in intriguing ways. Men's bodies maintain higher levels of neutrophils, the first responders of our immune system, well into their sixties. While they may face more frequent immune challenges, their systems often mount more robust acute responses when confronted with threats.

Research shows that men experience a 1.5 times faster decrease in brain volume, particularly in regions controlling memory and emotion. At the same time, women face their own distinct challenges with hormonal fluctuations that can affect cognitive processing and emotional regulation. These aren't mere statistics. They are doorways to understanding how our biological blueprints, unique to each sex, demand different attention as we move through our Second Prime.

The wisdom lies not in comparing patterns between sexes, but in recognizing how to work in harmony with our body's inherent nature. For example, a man in his sixties might notice that while a challenging hike brings more fatigue than it once did, his body still maintains its remarkable ability to repair and adapt when given the recovery time. These patterns become our guides, showing us when to pursue challenges and when to embrace recovery without guilt, shame, or disappointment in ourselves. In this light, choosing a health-focused life isn't merely preventive medicine. It's an acknowledgment of our changing biology and an intelligent response to what our bodies are telling us. Understanding these natural rhythms transforms aging from something that happens to us into a journey we actively shape, each sex dancing to its own unique but equally valuable biological dance party of one.

Similarly, a woman might find that while her processing speed for complex tasks may require more time, her enhanced verbal memory—that remarkable ability to recall conversations, stories, and life's narrative details with vivid clarity—combined with heightened emotional intelligence, allows her to navigate challenging situations with newfound depth and nuance. For example, when a daughter calls seeking advice about a workplace challenge, or a friend needs someone to truly hear their journey through grief, this capacity for verbal recall becomes more than a cognitive skill. It transforms into a bridge of understanding, allowing us to draw upon similar situations, remembered conversations, and hard-won wisdom to offer genuine insight and support.

The architecture of human connection reveals itself not through abstract numbers but through the careful observation of lives unfolding over time. The Harvard Study of Adult Development, the longest-running longitudinal study on aging and well-being, illuminates a profound truth. The warmth of human bonds protects our hearts and our very biology. Their findings show that people who are more socially connected to family, friends, and community are happier, physically healthier, and live longer than people who are less connected. The quality of close relationships at age fifty better predicted physical health than cholesterol levels.

The Nurses' Health Study, following more than ninety thousand women for over thirty years, discovered that women who were socially isolated faced health risks comparable to those from obesity and smoking. For men, the story echoes with equal significance. The *European Heart Journal* published findings that men with strong social connections showed markedly better recovery rates from heart attacks and significantly lower risks of recurring cardiac events.

This is the profound impact of every coffee shared with an old friend, every deep conversation that stretches into the evening, every moment of genuine connection that we might otherwise take for granted. As we explored earlier in our journey through this book, these bonds form the invisible architecture of our resilience, becoming increasingly vital as we navigate our Second Prime. Every genuine laugh shared, every vulnerability expressed, and every moment of being truly seen and understood becomes a social pleasure and a powerful investment in our quality of life and longevity.

The biology of aging isn't your destiny—it's your starting point. It's time that you honor your unique path through the Second Prime. Understanding sex differences isn't about accepting limitations but making informed choices and challenging unproductive norms. This journey invites intellectual curiosity as you become a fully integrated human in coherence, where your body's wisdom and your mind's understanding work as allies rather than adversaries.

True coherence happens when you stop treating yourself like a collection of disconnected parts. It's that "aha!" moment when your cells and neurons finally have a proper conversation after decades of awkward small talk. Think of it as your body's systems finally getting on the same Zoom call after years of sending passive-aggressive emails.

Your biological imperatives and conscious aspirations need

to shake hands and agree on a plan. When they do, you access dimensions of yourself that have been waiting in the wings, ready for their moment to shine in this brilliant second act of your life.

For women, biological advantages in aging are real but not guaranteed, like having a good hand in poker that still needs to be played well. Our natural tendency toward social connection and companionship isn't just nice to have; it's literally extending our lives. And while society actually supports our vulnerability and community-building, these connections aren't just pleasant social norms—they're powerful wellness strategies we can intentionally cultivate as we age.

Biological challenges for men as they age are not obstacles; they're invitations and opportunities to pioneer new ways of being, a new definition of being male, and a courageous openness that can reshape and sustain health, cognitive reserve, and the cardiovascular system. When you learn that emotional expression can reduce stress hormone levels by 23 percent, it becomes clear that vulnerability isn't weakness. It's a powerful tool for longevity and connection, as well as deeper and more meaningful relationships.

The most remarkable finding I've encountered is this: Up to 90 percent of our genes can be influenced by our lifestyle choices. Think about that for a moment. Your biological inheritance is just the opening chapter. You get to write the rest of the story.

Let me share something that changed my perspective entirely. During a workshop I led on aging, a successful businessman in his seventies stood up and said something I'll never forget: "I spent fifty years believing strength meant silence. Now I understand that my greatest strength is letting others hear my story."

Think of your social connections as a living infrastructure supporting your journey through the Second Prime. Women typically excel at maintaining these networks. Studies show they're three times more likely to seek emotional support with a friend or mental health professional during life transitions. But what is encouraging is that when men consciously cultivate strong friendships, they experience comparable longevity and cognitive health benefits.

A retired architect described it perfectly: "I used to think my weekly coffee dates with friends were just normal socializing. Now I understand I'm building the foundation for my future health." He's right. Research consistently shows that strong social networks significantly reduce the risk of cognitive decline across genders. The Lancet Commission on Dementia Prevention identifies social isolation as one of the top five modifiable risk factors for cognitive health in older adults.

The biological differences between men and women in aging aren't barriers; they're guideposts. They point us toward the areas where we can make the most impactful changes.

For women, your path might include:

- Leveraging your natural tendency toward social connection by creating intentional communities that support your growth and future plans.

- Understanding that your stronger verbal memory that comes with aging isn't just a gift. It's a tool for maintaining cognitive vitality.

- Recognizing that your extended life expectancy isn't guaranteed but can be enhanced through conscious choices and making time to pursue your inconvenient dream.

For men, this might mean:

- Challenging traditional narratives about emotional expression. Feel your feelings and share them.

- Creating new rituals of connection that feel authentic to you and those you love. Understand that your biological vulnerabilities can be offset through proactive health choices; spending time with others is an easy and fun way to promote your health.

- Schedule activity-based connection where you can use your hands or play a sport.

Remember Michael, the executive I mentioned earlier? Six months after our conversation, he discovered a profound truth disguised as a simple activity—walking.

"It's not therapy," he told me, laughing. Still, his eyes held the wisdom of someone who had stumbled upon something transformative. "My friends and I, we just talk about life while we walk. But somehow, it's changing everything; tough topics come naturally, and we have the opportunity to help and even heal one another."

What Michael discovered reflects a fundamental truth about masculine connection—the power of parallel activity. When men move together, whether walking shoulder to shoulder or sharing a task, the pressure of face-to-face vulnerability dissolves. The rhythm of footsteps and the shared pace create a natural space for conversation. This isn't just about exercise; it's about how movement liberates the voice and how physical activity provides the perfect cover for emotional exposure. Their walking group has become a master class in aging well, combining cardiovascular health, balance maintenance, and social connection, all while creating the conditions for meaningful male bonding that research shows is crucial for longevity.

What's fascinating is how this mirrors childhood's purest friendships before societal expectations layered shame onto male emotional intimacy. The Harvard Study of Adult Development has shown that social connection is far more important for health and longevity than many other factors, and movement-based activities can significantly facilitate these vital social bonds. This effect appears particularly pronounced for men, who often find it easier to engage in meaningful conversation during parallel activities than in face-to-face settings.

While women often excel at face-to-face connection, many also find that walking conversations unlock more profound sharing layers. One research participant noted, "Something about moving forward together makes it easier to move forward in our stories." This natural rhythm of walking and talking, this dance of connection through motion, reminds us that sometimes the most profound bonds emerge not from sitting still but from the simple act of moving forward together, step by step, story by story.

With each choice, we're not just drafting our story; we're influencing how our genes express themselves, how our telomeres protect our cellular health, how our neural pathways adapt and grow. May you look back at this moment and recognize it as one of those quiet turning points, where understanding transformed into action, where science became story.

Science offers us this remarkable truth: While our chromosomes may set the stage, they don't write the script. Whether through the quiet power of connection (which influences health more than cholesterol levels) or through reimagining what's possible at every age, your daily decisions actively shape your biology. Your body carries wisdom; honor it, but never let it become your boundary. The transformative power lies not in fighting nature but in making informed choices about how you want to dance with it.

Challenge: The Seven-Day Story Shift

Life whispers its wisdom to us in unexpected moments, through the quiet acknowledgment of a changing reflection, in the steady rhythm of our daily choices, in the gentle recognition of patterns we've inherited about how we should age. This week, I invite you to listen more deeply to these whispers and begin writing a new story about your journey through time.

Choose one simple action each day:

- **Day 1:** Notice one inherited belief about how someone of your gender "should" age. Observe it without judgment.

- **Day 2:** Challenge that belief through a tiny action. If you're a man who believes vulnerability shows weakness, share something meaningful with a friend. If you're a woman who feels pressure to hide signs of aging, celebrate one way your experience shows in your face or body.

- **Days 3–6:** Each day, take one action that honors your body's wisdom while gently pushing beyond gender expectations. This might be as simple as scheduling a health check-up you've been postponing, reaching out to deepen a friendship, or permitting yourself to rest without guilt. A few examples:

  - Take one story from your rich bank of memories each week and share it—by phone, in person, or even in a letter—with someone who played a part in it. Let the telling be a bridge to a deeper connection.

  - Share one thing that challenged you this week during your regular routines, perhaps a morning coffee with friends or an evening walk. Simple, direct, honest. Let this small opening create space for a natural connection.

- **Day 7:** Write a brief letter to your future self (see the following template), describing the aging story you choose to live beyond the constraints of aging and gender expectations discussed in the chapter.

A Letter to My Future Self: Honoring Nature's Wisdom

Dear Future Self,

In this moment of quiet reflection, I'm writing to you from the threshold of understanding—where science meets story, where biology meets becoming. Research tells us that up to 90 percent of our genetic expression is influenced by our daily choices. What a profound invitation to shape our own story!

Habits I Choose to Nurture: [Consider practices that honor your body's natural rhythms and strengths]

1. _____

2. _____

3. _____

4. _____

Patterns Ready to Transform: [Notice which cultural expectations no longer serve your evolution]

1. _____

2. _____

3. _____

Connection Rituals to Cultivate: [Remember: strong social bonds reduce cognitive decline by 43 percent]

1. _____

2. _____

3. _____

Relationships to Tend: [The Harvard Study reminds us: quality relationships predict health better than cholesterol levels]

1. _____

2. _____

Inconvenient Dreams to Pursue: [What story of aging are you ready to write?]

_____

_____

A Gift to My Future: [A specific intention that honors both biology and aspiration]

_____

_____

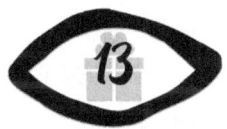

Pretty Rebellious: The Revolution Against Age-Based Beauty

The Roman poet Ovid called it two millennia ago: Is your own Narcissus in the mirror? This provocative question opens our exploration into the myth of Narcissus as it intersects with our modern world. Ovid, an expert storyteller and keen observer of human nature, wove this cautionary tale into his masterwork *Metamorphoses* around 8 CE. With his clever prose, ancient myths became mirrors reflecting timeless truths about our mortal character, desire, and transformation. Ovid understood something profound about our relationship with beauty and self-image, insights that echo hauntingly through the ether of our culture today.

In Ovid's telling, Narcissus was born to the female deity river nymph Liriope, who received a prophecy about her son's fate: He would live a long life, provided he never came to know himself. This cryptic warning unfolds in the story of a youth blessed with such extraordinary beauty that all who beheld him fell deeply in love. Yet Narcissus met his admirer's devotion with cold disdain. When the nymph Echo fell hopelessly in love with him, he rejected her with cruel indifference, leaving her to fade away until only her voice remained eternally repeating the last words of others. His punishment came through divine justice. Upon seeing his reflection in a clear pool, he fell hopelessly in love with his image. Unable to tear himself away from this illusory love, he gradually withered, transforming in death into the flower that bears his name—a beautiful bloom that still nods perpetually downward as if gazing at its reflection in the water below.

Fast forward and one can't help but see the ripples of this narrative in our selfie-obsessed society. Are we not, like Narcissus, entranced by our own reflections and then, as we age, repelled by them? Do we risk drowning in the shallow pools of superficiality? The quest for eternal youth and flawless beauty often eclipses our more profound worth, confining us to a realm where our value is measured by our reflection—our followers, likes, and shares.

The act of taking selfies or capturing our own images speaks to the fundamental human desire to see ourselves, to be seen, and to leave our mark (although it does make me cringe at times). Social media and self-documentation can be a vehicle for creativity, a conduit for connection, and a testament to our existence in a rapidly evolving world. Yet, I challenge us to look beyond the surface and question what these reflections stand for.

Picture a social media platform that pulses with the rhythm of real lives. Not just carefully curated moments, but the full spectrum of human experience across generations. Here's how we might reimagine this digital landscape.

Imagine a space where a teenager's exuberant selfie sits alongside her grandmother's photo from 1975, both celebrations of their respective moments in time. But beneath these images lies something more profound, stories that weave together the timeless pursuit of self-discovery. The platform encourages users to pair images with reflections. "What made you feel beautiful today?" or "Share a moment when you felt truly seen."

The architecture of this space would deliberately blur the lines between generations, creating what we might call beauty bridges: digital gathering places where a sixteen-year-old's passion for makeup artistry can coexist with a sixty-year-old's journey of embracing her silver hair. Both stories hold equal weight, teaching the other something vital about beauty and self-expression.

Instead of algorithms that reinforce narrow beauty standards, imagine a system that rewards authenticity and cross-generational dialogue. A young influencer's post about her latest skincare routine might automatically link to wisdom from older users about self-acceptance, creating a natural flow between the celebration of youth and appreciation of aging.

The platform could feature timeline treasures, paired stories where users of different ages share parallel moments in their beauty journeys. A teenager wrestling with acne might find unexpected kinship with a woman in her fifties navigating wrinkles, learning that our relationship with our reflection is less about perfection and more about perspective.

This isn't about dismissing young people's natural desire to explore and express through appearance, nor is it about diminishing older individuals' right to care about how they look. Rather, it's about creating a space where every age can recognize beauty as a form of self-expression rather than a standard to achieve.

Think of it as a digital safe space where the pressure to be perfect gradually dissolves into the joy of being present. Where each generation learns from the others that beauty isn't a destination but a journey of becoming. Here, social media transforms from a mirror that demands perfection into a window that reveals our shared humanity across all ages and stages.

What could emerge is not just a platform but a new way of seeing, one that teaches us all—regardless of age—that our worth isn't measured in likes but discovered in the courage to be authentically ourselves at every stage of life.

Throughout history, our relationship with our reflection has evolved from those first glimpses in still pools of water to today's endless stream of digital mirrors. Each era brought its own standards of beauty and its own ways of measuring worth. Still, none has been as relentless as our current age of constant documentation and comparison. In this chapter, let's confront these questions head-on by delving into the historical context of beauty, value, and age that has influenced much of the social and self-perception of growing older.

The world has convinced women that our value is primarily measured by the firmness of our skin, the brightness of our smile, or the size of our waistline. It's time to shatter this mirror of deception that limits our future selves. Like the polished bronze mirrors of ancient civilizations that showed imperfect reflections, perhaps our modern mirrors—both physical and digital—are equally distorted by societal expectations and internalized prejudices.

Imagine if Narcissus had looked beyond the surface. If he had seen the depth of his soul rather than the impermanence and shallowness of his appearance. What if he had recognized that the pool reflected only the most superficial aspect of his being? Modern humans face a similar challenge—to see beyond the reflecting glass that society holds up to us, to recognize our worth in the depths rather than the surface.

As we move into our Second Prime, women experience what they've learned from birth; youth and beauty go hand in hand. The relentless pressure of society's physical standards carves a deep chasm between the aging experience of men and women. A man is depicted as aging like a fine wine, his graying hair a crown of wisdom, his weathered face a map of journeys taken, each wrinkle a badge of honor. These signs of aging may be viewed with reverence as indicators of a distinguished, seasoned life. This is the chiseled picture of the silver fox in his Second Prime.

Women stand on the other side of this chasm, facing expectations that defy nature. Like a flower expected to remain in perpetual bloom, we confront an unwavering pressure to retain our youthfulness. The concept of beauty continues its eternal dance of transformation, ever-changing. From the curvaceous pin-up girls of the 1950s, through the Twiggy-inspired waifs of the sixties, to the fitness-obsessed supermodels of the 1980s, we've witnessed countless iterations of the ideal. Today's more diverse representations offer hope, yet the underlying message persists: youth equals value.

Yet there is hope. An excellent example of changing norms is the body-positivity revolution, which is reshaping our cultural landscape through deliberate, strategic action. Like a wave gathering force, it began with advocates demanding change where it mattered most: store windows sprouting diverse mannequins, fashion campaigns featuring varied bodies, social media feeds highlighting authentic lives. The impact of inclusive representation has been measurable, a win for inclusivity. After Target introduced diverse mannequins in 2016, customer satisfaction scores increased by 24 percent among women shoppers. Also in 2016, *Sports Illustrated* featured Ashley Graham, their first-ever plus-sized cover model for the swimsuit issue and saw newsstand sales increase by 15 percent compared to the previous year. The Dove "Real Beauty" campaign launched in 2004, which featured women of diverse body types, helped increase Dove's sales from $2.5 billion to $4 billion in the campaign's first ten years.

Now imagine this same transformative energy directed at ageism. Just as we rewrote the rules about body diversity, we can challenge our youth-obsessed culture's narrow definition of beauty. The blueprint exists for coordinated pressure that makes age diversity not just culturally vital but economically smart. What if beauty campaigns featured women in their Second Prime not as tokens but as standard-bearers? What if we transformed anti-aging into pro-living, celebrating each line and silver hair as evidence of a life richly lived?

This isn't just about changing what we see in mirrors and magazines. It's about expanding society's vision of what makes a life beautiful. The body-positivity movement showed us that cultural norms bend when enough voices demand change. Now it's time to apply these tested strategies to age, making space for every chapter of our story to be seen, honored, and celebrated.

Our language becomes the lens through which we view ourselves and others. A depressing study from Dove revealed that only 4 percent of women worldwide consider themselves beautiful, a statistic that echoes in our daily conversations, in those seemingly innocent qualifiers that carry the weight of judgment: "She's pretty . . . for her age." "She looks great . . . considering." These verbal asterisks we attach to compliments become tiny paper cuts to our collective self-worth, reinforcing the idea that beauty has an expiration date.

Listen to how we speak about ourselves and each other. The casual self-deprecation, the apologetic tone when we admit our age, and the way we preface compliments with conditions that diminish their power. This isn't just semantics. It's the architecture of our self-image, built word by careful word. When we qualify beauty with age, we tacitly agree that youth is the standard against which all beauty must be measured.

But what if we consciously shifted this ageist narrative? Imagine complimenting a woman's radiant smile without adding "for her age" or celebrating her vibrant energy without the caveat of "despite being in her forties." What if we spoke about ourselves and others with words that honor rather than apologize for the passage of time? "She's stunning." Full stop. "Her presence fills the room." "She is so witty!" No qualifiers needed. "I love how my experience shows in my face." Period.

This isn't just about positive thinking. It's about dismantling the linguistic scaffolding that supports ageism. Every time we catch ourselves adding those qualifying phrases, we have an opportunity to rewrite the script. In this way, our daily conversations become small but powerful acts of revolution, each unqualified compliment a brick removed from the wall of age-based beauty standards.

This pressure placed on women is enormous and transforms time into a countdown clock, marking the journey from visibility to what many women describe as a kind of social invisibility. A landmark 2019 study by the University of Melbourne, surveying over two thousand women aged forty to seventy-five, revealed that the experience of social invisibility begins to peak in women's mid-fifties, with significant impacts on their professional and personal lives. The research showed that while 78 percent of women under forty-five reported feeling "seen" in professional settings, this dropped to just 43 percent in the fifty-five to sixty-five age group.

The experience of invisibility manifests in layers. Think of how a woman moves through the world in her younger years, existing in a constant state of awareness, like an actress on a perpetually lit stage. The ambient hum of male attention forms the background music of daily life: appreciative glances, held doors, eager smiles, and conversations that bloom quickly in elevators and coffee shops. While this attention can be unwanted and sometimes threatening, its presence shapes how she navigates her world, creating a particular kind of visibility that you don't fully notice until it's gone.

Then comes the shift, unfolding like a slow-motion disappearing act. In professional settings, it manifests as being passed over for leadership roles or having expertise questioned more frequently. Conversations in meetings flow around her like water around a stone. In restaurants, the server's eyes drift past to younger patrons. Male gazes, once a constant companion whether welcomed or not, begin to slide away, drawn to younger faces like moths to brighter flames. She finds herself standing in a curious new space, neither here nor there, as if existing in the margins of society's attention.

This feeling of invisibility arrives bearing gifts and grievances, like a mysterious package containing loss and liberation. Some women speak of mourning their visible selves, missing the social currency that came with being seen as young or conventionally attractive. The absence of male attention becomes a mirror reflecting our society's more profound beliefs about women's value, raising uncomfortable questions. How much of our sense of self-worth has been unconsciously tied to male validation? How do we navigate this transition when our culture offers so few models of women aging powerfully rather than apologetically?

Yet others describe a profound sense of freedom, like finally being released from an exhausting performance they didn't realize they'd been giving their entire lives. In social situations, even as they notice the subtle shift in how others direct their attention, they discover a new kind of presence, one built not on being seen but on seeing clearly for perhaps the first time.

The transformation comes when we realize that true visibility isn't about being seen by others but about finally seeing ourselves clearly, free from the distorting lens of external validation. Perhaps this is the most powerful revelation of our Second Prime: We can exist beyond the boundaries of society's gaze, defining our presence not by who notices us but by how fully we inhabit our own lives.

In this light, our relationship with visibility evolves into something more nuanced and profound. The same woman who might be overlooked in a restaurant could be simultaneously discovering her most authentic voice, leading with wisdom rather than appearance, and finding power in the invisibility that once threatened to diminish her. She learns that being seen isn't the same as being known, and that the most valuable recognition comes from within.

This journey through the territory of Second Prime becomes

not just a personal transformation but a radical redefinition of worth. It suggests that our value isn't measured in admiring glances or social currency, but in the courage to pursue those inconvenient dreams that have waited patiently for their moment. The fading of one kind of visibility becomes an invitation to step into a more authentic way of being seen not just by others, but by ourselves.

In this way, what society might frame as a loss of relevance becomes instead a gateway to the significance of a different kind. One measured not in youthful beauty but in the profound impact of living true to our calling, whatever form that might take.

From Egyptian queens adorning themselves with golden beads to medieval women risking their health with lead-based powders, the worship of youth stretches back through centuries. It's not a product of modern media but a deeper cultural narrative that has insisted, generation after generation, that women occupy an impossible space. Be beautiful, but make it look effortless. Age gracefully, but don't age at all. This emphasis has profoundly shaped our understanding of femininity and womanhood, inter-twining our sense of value with our reflection in ways that deserve careful unraveling.

The indoctrination begins early, woven into the fabric of our childhood stories. In 1812, when the Brothers Grimm first pub-lished "Snow White," they crystallized in print a tale that would echo through generations, embedding itself in our cultural DNA. What began as a German fairy tale soon transcended borders and languages, becoming a universal parable about youth, beauty, and the perceived tragedy of aging. Through countless retellings and Disney's technicolor dreams, this story has shaped how we view the journey of female aging, casting long shadows that still darken our relationship with time.

At its heart lies the aging queen, tormented by her mirror's daily judgment, a reflection not just of her fading youth but of society's persistent equation of beauty with worth. For over two centuries, this narrative has taught young girls to fear their own future, to view older women as cautionary tales rather than guides, and to see aging as a kind of failure rather than a triumph of experience.

Yet, in recognizing how deeply these narratives have shaped us since that first publication, we gain the power to question them. Perhaps it's time to retell this two-hundred-year-old story, not through the lens of fear and competition but through the wisdom of women stepping confidently into their Second Prime. In this version, beauty and worth are measured not by a mirror's shallow reflection but by the depth of life's well-earned stories.

Each morning, countless women stand before mirrors, engaging in that intimate ritual of self-reflection that carries far more weight than simply applying moisturizer or choosing an outfit. The beauty industry, worth over five hundred billion dollars globally, promotes eternal youth while the wisdom of our Second Prime whispers of something far more valuable. As we transition into our Second Prime, there is grief and loss for what was. This transition, if not acknowledged and honored, can become a source of shame.

Yet within this very challenge lies our Second Prime invitation to commemorate our progress into a new phase of life with more depth and growth than we have previously understood. When studies show that women in their later years often report feeling more confident and self-assured than in their youth, we glimpse a profound truth—aging brings challenges and unexpected liberation. It's the ideal time to redefine beauty on our own terms and recognize that the more we embody our authentic selves, the more we grow in mastery of life. This isn't about rejecting beauty or self-care; it's about expanding the definition of what makes a life beautiful. Some days, that might mean an hour at the salon that helps us feel refreshed and confident. Other days, it might mean skipping makeup entirely to focus on launching a new project that sets our soul on fire.

Beauty standards constantly evolve, yet the veneration of youth remains steadfast, like an ancient ritual we've forgotten to question. This can make navigating the physical aging process difficult for even the most centered and grounded women. We face unique challenges in our journey, confronting society's uncomfortable silence around mature sexuality and the profound transitions of menopause, powerful shifts that mark not an ending but a transformation into our next chapter.

Like many shadowed aspects of women's experience, menopause has long been whispered about behind closed doors. Yet today, we witness a remarkable shift. What was once taboo has emerged into the light, becoming a burgeoning market with a multitude of products and services to support the menopausal journey. The open conversation is a real-time evolution showing us something profound about the nature of change. Shame can dissolve when we dare to speak our truth aloud; the shadow of aging recedes when we shine a light on our shared experiences. This is the blueprint for a more significant transformation, showing us how every aspect of aging that society has taught us to fear can become instead a catalyst for liberation and authentic expression.

The media's portrayal of aging women reveals our culture's complex and often contradictory relationship with female aging. While recent years have witnessed breakthrough moments— celebrated actresses over fifty commanding lead roles, streaming series exploring women's later-life adventures, and advertising campaigns featuring silver-haired models—these changes ripple across the surface of more profound, more resistant currents. Like stars appearing in a gradually darkening sky, these representations, though bright and hopeful, have yet to fully illuminate the landscape.

Primetime television still tells a revealing story. Female characters consistently appear younger than their male counterparts, while older women often find themselves confined to the margins of the narrative, their roles as narrow as the beauty standards they're expected to maintain. For every Helen Mirren or Viola Davis breaking new ground, countless talented mature actresses face a drought of meaningful opportunities. Meanwhile, men gracefully transition into roles of distinguished wizards and elder statesmen, their age adding to their authenticity and authority rather than being a mark of irrelevance.

As examined in our exploration of marketing and perception, these representations aren't merely reflections; they're architects of cultural attitudes, shaping how society views aging women and how we view ourselves. While worth celebrating, the occasional breakthrough shouldn't lull us into complacency. Rather, it should illuminate the path toward a media landscape where women of all ages see themselves not as stereotypes but as the complex, vibrant beings we truly are.

Our Second Prime offers us not just years of experience, but the wisdom to recognize that beauty flows from purpose, from the courage to pursue our inconvenient dreams to the authenticity of finally releasing society's restrictive expectations. Each line on our face maps a journey taken, and each silver strand marks a battle won or lesson learned. These are not flaws to be erased but a testament to lives fully lived, which is incredibly beautiful!

Challenge: Look for the Beauty Within

Embracing your radiant Second Prime, consider this not just a set of questions but an invitation to transformation. Like those pivotal moments that reshape our understanding of ourselves, each reflection offers a chance to rewrite the narrative of aging and beauty.

Have you ever noticed how certain people draw you in at a soul level? While their appearance might create an initial spark, it's their essence, their authentic being, that truly captivates. This is your invitation to shift focus from the mirror to the heart to the energy you exude, from surface to substance. Research shows that when women focus on purpose over appearance, their reported life satisfaction increases significantly.

Consider

- What are the top five qualities you find uniquely beautiful in others?

- In what ways might redirecting your energy from scrutinizing perceived imperfections toward nurturing these soul-deep virtues transform both your inner landscape and your outward presence in the world?

- Which campaigns or movements have helped you recognize your innate value beyond physical attributes?

- How has seeing positive representations of women in their Second Prime influenced your journey?

Challenge the Norms

- What are some ways you can dismantle societal norms equating a woman's worth with her physical beauty and youth?

- Do you challenge ageist language when you meet it?

- Can you think of ways to introduce positive age inclusive comments into your everyday conversations?

Food for Thought

- Where have you seen successful campaigns or movements that have redefined public feeling, promoting a more inclusive definition of beauty? How do these campaigns reassure you of your innate value?

- How can you make it your own personal campaign to incorporate positive internal messaging and curb negative self-talk?

- What nurturing practices do you use to rewire your neurons in a positive way? What feelings do you notice when you do these practices?

Redefine Beauty Talks

- How do you engage in discussions about beauty and skincare with friends? How can you use language that supports self-care versus self-criticism?

- How can you be the one to break the cycle? How can you choose to see the beauty in all humans?

- How can you encourage younger people within your influence to redefine how they view beauty?

Find Your Role Models

- List five to ten women who embody the positive ideals of embracing their Second Prime. What is it about them that gains your admiration?

- How can you apply their lifestyles and experiences as inspiration to redefine your own narrative of beauty and aging?

- How can you strive to become a positive aging role model for others?

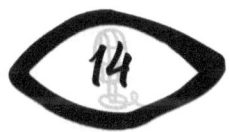

The Power of Three: Autonomy, Agency, and the Art of Optimistic Living

Life often surprises us with moments that transform how we see ourselves. A friend's mother comes to mind. After decades of marriage, she found herself widowed and facing a startling realization: She had no idea how to access their joint accounts, manage their investments, or even oversee fundamental household decisions her husband had always seen to. Her story is a simple yet consistent reminder that independence isn't just about making choices; it's about maintaining the desire and capacity to make them.

Her story illustrates what I've heard countless times in different variations while researching for this book. This is the quiet revelation that somewhere along the way, we've unconsciously surrendered pieces of our autonomy, one small decision at a time. Sometimes, these moments arrive like thunderclaps, impossible to ignore. More often, they sidle up to us in the quiet hours, gentle nudges that something in our lives has shifted out of alignment. It's in these moments that we often find the first hints that we've allowed our personal power to slowly erode, like water wearing away at the stone.

The timing of this awakening varies for each of us. Some recognize it in their thirties when they realize they've built a life to please others rather than themselves. Others encounter it in midlife, questioning the automatic patterns that have governed their decisions. Still others face it in their later years, confronting the cumulative effect of delegated choices. What matters isn't when this recognition comes but what we choose to do with it.

Consider Leigh, who at thirty-five found herself standing in her corner office, surrounded by the trappings of what society deemed successful. She had the prestigious law degree, the partnership track position, the carefully curated wardrobe that projected authority. Her days were mapped out in fifteen-minute increments, each hour a testament to efficiency and ambition. Yet in quiet moments, when the office grew still, she felt the weight of choices made through the lens of others' expectations.

She had followed the prescribed path with precision, attending a top-tier university, landing competitive internships, making herself visible at strategic networking events. Each step was carefully chosen not from inner conviction, but from an inherited blueprint of success. The revelation came not in a dramatic moment of crisis, but in the gentle understanding that her childhood dream of opening a community bookstore—dismissed years ago as impractical—still whispered to her soul with surprising persistence.

Autonomy, agency, and optimism form a potent blend of inner resources that significantly influence our journey through aging, especially during our Second Prime. These intertwined qualities create a dynamic empowerment triad that amplifies our well-being, fortifies our resilience, and shapes the very architecture of our later years. They are not merely complementary forces; they are the three pillars upon which we build a life of meaning and purpose, each strengthening and supporting the others in a continuous dance of personal empowerment.

When these characteristics are authentically integrated into our lives, they support our physiological health in ways that science is only beginning to fully understand. They influence our epigenetics—the intricate symphony of gene expression that responds to our daily choices and experiences. Think of your genes not as a rigid blueprint but as a responsive musical score, where your life-style choices serve as the conductor determining which notes are played loudly and which remain silent.

Recent research in epigenetics reveals how our mental and emotional states can directly reshape our biological narrative. When we exercise autonomy and agency, supported by an optimistic outlook, we trigger beneficial changes in gene expression that affect everything from inflammation levels to cellular aging. It's as if each empowered decision, each moment of conscious choice, and each optimistic perspective send a ripple through our biological system, influencing which genes are activated and which remain dormant.

Studies show that individuals who maintain control over their lives (autonomy) typically display more favorable gene expression patterns related to inflammation and immune function. Those who actively engage in life-directing behaviors (agency) show improved markers for cellular repair and stress resistance. And perhaps most fascinating, research indicates that an optimistic outlook is associated with patterns of gene expression that enhance longevity and resilience at the cellular level.

This conversation between our choices and our cells subtly and profoundly writes its signature on our biological story. Every time we choose to exercise our autonomy, engage our agency, or maintain our optimism, we're not just making a mental choice—we're orchestrating a complex biological response that can influence our health trajectory. It's a testament to the remarkable plasticity of our bodies and the power we hold to affect our biology through the choices we make and the attitudes we cultivate.

In an ideal world, we'd live unbound by external constraints, reveling in our emotional and societal freedoms, fully expressing our true selves. We'd naturally build the life we envision. But the reality is more complex, more nuanced. We all live under a web of constraints that shape our choices and limit our movements, often in ways we've stopped noticing.

Some constraints are apparent, such as governmental policies that affect our healthcare choices, societal norms that dictate "appropriate" behavior for our age or gender, or financial systems that may have left us behind. Others are woven into the fabric of our daily lives, like the subtle dynamics of an unequal marriage where one partner holds the financial reins, the well-meaning family members who've gradually taken over decision-making "for our own good," or the community expectations that silently pressure us to conform rather than evolve.

These invisible bonds of control weave themselves so gradually into our lives that their presence often goes unnoticed until they've formed an intricate web of constraint. Consider how financial dependency in relationships creates a power dynamic that extends far beyond merely who pays the bills. It shapes daily choices, from the seemingly trivial decision about ordering dessert to the profound question of pursuing a career change. Studies suggest that women in financially dependent relationships are 50 percent more likely to experience depression and anxiety, highlighting the profound psychological impact of diminished autonomy.

Religious communities, while offering valuable support and belonging, can unconsciously restrict personal growth through unspoken rules and expectations. The pressure to maintain appearances, attend certain events, or raise children according to specific doctrines can slowly eclipse individual spiritual journeys. This social pressure often manifests in physical symptoms. Studies have linked religious strain to increased cortisol levels and compromised immune function.

Perhaps most insidious are the societal structures that limit reproductive autonomy. When access to healthcare becomes entangled with political ideology, the impact ripples through every aspect of life—career choices, relationship dynamics, and mental well-being. Research has shown that women living in areas with restricted reproductive rights report higher levels of chronic stress and delayed medical care across all health needs, not just reproductive services.

These constraints compound quietly, like sediment building up in a river, gradually narrowing its flow. A mother postpones her education to meet family expectations, a spouse silences their career aspirations to maintain domestic harmony, and a teenager suppresses their identity to fit community norms. Each compromise seems small in isolation, but together, they form a dam against authentic self-expression and well-being.

The toll isn't just emotional. It manifests in our bodies through elevated stress hormones, disrupted sleep patterns, and compromised immune responses. According to recent health studies, chronic stress from sustained loss of autonomy can accelerate cellular aging and increase susceptibility to various health conditions.

After fifteen years of marriage, my dear friend Katie realized that she had never really chosen where to go on vacation—her husband always made those decisions. Then there's James, who discovered that his children had begun making medical appointments for him without consultation, slowly eroding his sense of agency over his own healthcare. These constraints don't announce themselves with fanfare; they creep in on little cat paws, becoming our normal before we've had a chance to question them.

Yet perhaps the most challenging limitations are the ones we place upon ourselves, the invisible fences we erect around our possibilities, often without conscious awareness. These self-imposed boundaries become so familiar that we mistake them for immutable truths rather than the malleable stories they genuinely are.

Autonomy, agency, and optimism aren't merely beneficial

qualities to cultivate. They are essential life-enriching forces that deserve the same careful attention we give to nourishing our bodies and minds. Together, they form the foundation of sustainable independence—the ability to maintain control over our lives even as circumstances change.

Research reveals a fascinating synergy between these three elements. A groundbreaking study from the *Journal of Personality and Social Psychology* demonstrated that individuals with higher levels of optimism were more likely to take active steps toward maintaining their autonomy. At the same time, those who exercised greater agency naturally developed more optimistic outlooks. It's a virtuous cycle. Each element strengthens the others, creating an upward spiral of empowerment.

At its core, autonomy is about more than making independent decisions. It's about maintaining the sacred space of self-determination, protecting our right to author our own story. When we exercise autonomy, we're not just choosing what to do; we're choosing who to be.

Agency goes beyond simple action-taking. It's the profound recognition that we can be architects of change in our lives and that we possess the power to shape our circumstances rather than merely react to them. Through agency, we transform our inconvenient dreams from wistful possibilities into concrete realities.

Optimism, the third pillar of our empowerment triad, isn't about wearing rose-colored glasses or denying life's challenges. Instead, it's about maintaining a grounded belief in our capacity to navigate those challenges successfully. Research from the Yale School of Public Health shows that individuals with a more optimistic outlook have a higher survival rate of 11 to 15 percent, longer than their more pessimistic peers. This isn't just positive thinking. It's a practical tool for resilience and growth.

The power of these three elements working in concert cannot

be overstated. We're more likely to exercise our agency when we approach life's challenges optimistically. When we exercise our agency, we strengthen our autonomy. And when we experience the benefits of greater sovereignty, our optimism naturally grows. It's a self-reinforcing cycle that becomes stronger with each turn.

The research supporting the importance of these qualities is compelling. Studies consistently show that older adults who maintain their independence and actively exercise their sense of agency enjoy enhanced mental health, superior life satisfaction, and improved physical well-being. A landmark study in the *Journal of Aging and Health* revealed a fascinating correlation: Higher levels of perceived control were linked to better health outcomes and longer life spans.

Much like an architect plans a structure to withstand time and elements, we must consciously design our independence to be sustainable and resilient. This architecture begins with its most crucial element—decision fitness. Just as we exercise our bodies, we must consciously strengthen our decision-making muscles. This isn't about making perfect choices; it's about building the capability to make our own choices with increasing confidence and clarity.

Think of decision fitness like any other form of strength training. You begin where you are, gradually increasing the weight of decisions you carry. Start with small choices—where to go for dinner, what to wear, or how to spend your evening. Notice where you habitually defer to others' judgments. Each time you catch yourself automatically yielding your power, pause. Ask yourself: What would I choose if I fully trusted my own wisdom?

As your decision fitness grows, so does your capacity to manage weightier choices. Like muscle strengthening through consistent exercise, your ability to make autonomous decisions becomes more natural, more instinctive. The initial discomfort of claiming your choices gives way to a quiet confidence in your own judgment.

This foundation of decision fitness supports three essential pillars:

1. **The Foundation of Self-Trust:** Building on your growing decision fitness, deepen your connection to your own inner knowing. Notice the inner voice of your authentic preferences and the subtle nudges of your genuine desires. Let each small choice become a brick in the foundation of trusting yourself.

2. **The Framework of Capability:** Build your competence systematically across key life domains.

   - Financial sovereignty (understanding and managing your resources)
   - Health advocacy (being an active participant in your well-being)
   - Living arrangements (creating and maintaining your ideal environment)
   - Social connections (cultivating relationships that honor your autonomy)
   - Personal growth (continuously expanding your capabilities)

3. **The Support Structure:** Create a network of resources that enhances rather than diminishes your independence.

   - Professional advisors who respect your agency
   - Skills and knowledge that support self-reliance
   - Community connections that enrich without entangling
   - Technology tools that expand your capabilities

The science is clear. Those who maintain their autonomy and agency while nurturing optimistic perspectives experience better health outcomes, increased life satisfaction, and more vibrant engagement with life. But beyond the statistics lies a profound truth. The quality of our Second Prime depends largely on our willingness to claim and maintain our personal power.

Your future self is waiting, watching the choices you make today. Every small act of reclaimed autonomy, every moment of strengthened agency, every choice to maintain optimism in the face of challenge are the building blocks of a Second Prime that unfolds by design.

As we've explored the profound interplay between autonomy, agency, and optimism, we discovered that these forces shape more than our external reality. They coordinate an intricate dance within our very cells. Each empowered choice, each moment of conscious agency, ripples through our biological landscape like stones cast upon still waters. What science is now revealing about this mind-body connection extends far deeper than we once imagined, into an unexplored universe that exists within us all. A world where trillions of microscopic allies await our partnership, ready to transform our intentions into biological reality.

The journey into this hidden realm—our microbiome— reveals how the choices we make from this place of empowerment don't just change our story; they literally reshape our cellular narrative. As we step into this next exploration, we'll discover how the power to direct our lives extends into the very foundation of our physical being, where the smallest residents of our body stand ready to support our Second Prime transformation.

Challenge: The Thirty-Day Sovereignty Sprint

The journey to greater personal sovereignty begins with conscious awareness and deliberate action. Remember, this journey isn't about dramatic declarations of independence or severing connections. It's about consciously designing a life where our relationships enhance rather than override our autonomy, where your choices reflect our deepest values rather than unconscious patterns. Each day brings us closer to the fullest expression of who we're meant to be.

For the next thirty days, commit to this structured exploration of your autonomy and agency. End each day by writing in your journal or jotting a note on your phone:

- One decision I made entirely for myself today.
- One area where I noticed myself deferring unnecessarily.
- One step I took toward greater independence.

Week 1: Awareness

- Keep a daily log of decisions you make and decisions you defer.
- Note patterns of automatic yielding to others' preferences.
- Identify one small decision you'll reclaim each day.

Week 2: Capability Building

- Choose one life domain (financial, health, social, etc.).
- Learn one new skill in this domain.
- Practice making decisions in this area without seeking validation.

Week 3: Boundary Setting

- Identify relationships where your autonomy needs strengthening.

- Practice phrases that assert your agency: *I'll consider that and let you know my decision.*

- Notice and celebrate moments of standing in your power.

Week 4: Integration

- Review your progress and patterns.

- Strengthen areas where you've seen success.

- Plan your next focus area for continued growth.

Your Inner Pharmacy: Harnessing Microbiome Magic

Imagine a vast, unexplored wilderness teeming with life—an intricate ecosystem where countless species coexist, each vying for dominance, all while playing a vital role in maintaining balance and harmony. I'm not describing a distant rainforest or a deep-sea trench; it's the bustling world inside your body. Your microbiome is beyond astonishing. I call it your inner pharmacy, your biological frontier that holds the keys to health and the very essence of who you are now and your unfolding future self.

Within you lies an extraordinary marvel of evolution—a digestive tract that, if stretched end to end, would span approximately thirty feet. From the moment food enters your mouth until its final journey through the large intestine, this intricate system engineers a complex process of digestion, absorption, and transformation. What makes this system remarkable isn't just its length or complexity. It's the trillions of tiny inhabitants calling it home. In fact, the surface area of our gut—where these microorganisms reside— is roughly three thousand square feet, equivalent to a tennis court, providing an expansive playground for these beneficial beings.

Like an ancient forest adapting to an ever-changing climate, our microbiome shifts and evolves as we age. Around sixty years of age, our microbiome begins a delicate transition and change, its diversity gently declining like autumn leaves falling from a tree. Yet this natural shift isn't a diminishment. It's an invitation to deeper awareness and intentional nurturing and to pay more attention to how you tend to your inner pharmacy.

Our microbiome is an ancient teacher of resilience and a topic that could fill countless books. What we know is only overshadowed by what we have yet to discover. This microscopic universe, primarily housed in our gut, is home to trillions of microorganisms, including bacteria, viruses, fungi, and archaea. These last organisms—archaea—hold a special place in my heart because they embody everything we celebrate about the Second Prime journey. While humanity's story spans a mere fraction of Earth's history, archaea have been here since life's earliest moments, perfecting the art of adaptation across billions of years in the most challenging environments. In many ways, they are our most ancient teachers of resilience and transformation.

Archaea have not merely survived but thrived in conditions that would kill most organisms—from scalding hot springs to the depths of ocean trenches. These remarkable microorganisms perform crucial functions that science is only beginning to fully appreciate. They're the primary recyclers of our internal ecosystem, breaking down nutrients and producing essential compounds that support our cellular health. Like silent alchemists, they transform hydrogen and carbon dioxide into methane, helping maintain the delicate balance of our digestive system.

As we age, research suggests these resilient creatures face their own challenges, with their populations sometimes declining or shifting in composition. Yet true to their ancient nature, they adapt and persist. But we can support our remarkable residents in our biological community through mindful choices—maintaining a diverse diet rich in fiber, staying hydrated, and nurturing the very conditions that allow them to flourish.

Though our journey spans a much shorter timeframe, the resilience and adaptation of our microbiome is an example of what we're called to do in our Second Prime. Like these ancient microbes, we carry an innate wisdom that deepens with time, an ability to transform challenges into catalysts for growth, and a capacity to maintain our essential vitality even as conditions around us change. Just as archaea have survived multiple mass extinctions and continue to thrive in Earth's most extreme environments, we possess remarkable resilience. They remind us that adaptation isn't about dramatic transformations, but rather about finding innovative ways to remain fundamentally ourselves while meeting life's evolving challenges.

During early embryonic development, the same cluster of cells forms our central nervous system, which also gives rise to our enteric nervous system—our gut's neural network. Imagine these neurons stretching, reaching, and growing apart yet maintaining an intricate dialogue through the vagus nerve, our body's information superhighway. This isn't just fascinating embryology; it's the foundation of who we are. It reminds us that our gut and brain were never truly separate entities but rather two aspects of the same conscious system. It's a biological fact that the conversation between our gut and brain is non-stop and operates in tandem, sharing millions of bits of information a second.

This ancient wisdom takes on new meaning as we journey into our Second Prime. Research shows that our gut-brain axis actually becomes more refined with age, like a well-practiced duet. The phrase "listen to your gut" has roots in the Middle Ages, when people believed the gut was the seat of emotions and intuition—an ancestral knowing that modern science has now validated. You're likely familiar with the remarkable fact that 95 percent of your body's serotonin—often called the happiness molecule—is produced in your gut. Let that sink in for a moment: The very foundation of your emotional well-being is intimately tied to the health of your digestive system. This is why that morning coffee ritual, the comforting bowl of soup, or the fresh salad you enjoy doesn't just nourish your body. It literally shapes your emotional landscape.

A profound grace comes with aging, a deepening awareness of our body's subtle languages. Like an old friend whose gestures we've come to understand implicitly, our body speaks to us through whispers and signals that grow clearer with each passing year. This isn't just poetic musing. Research shows that older adults often demonstrate superior interoceptive awareness—the ability to sense and interpret internal bodily signals. What's particularly fascinating is that as we age, while our microbiome diversity may naturally decline, our gut's neural network maintains remarkable plasticity. Studies have shown that people over sixty who actively nurture their gut health through diet and lifestyle often demonstrate stronger gut-brain communication than their younger counterparts.

Think of it as your inner ecosystem gaining wisdom alongside you. Every probiotic-rich meal, every mindful moment, every conscious breath contributes to this profound internal conversation that's been developing since before your first heartbeat. Studies from the Human Microbiome Project reveal that older adults with more diverse gut bacteria often show better cognitive function and emotional resilience, suggesting that this deepening relationship with our body's intuition isn't just experiential. It's written into our very biology.

As we age, this intimate knowledge of our rhythms and responses becomes one of life's most valuable currencies. The subtle awareness of how certain foods affect our energy, how specific movements wake up our vitality, or how particular practices ground our nervous system aren't just random observations but a carefully curated wisdom library built through decades of living in our remarkable bodies. It's a kind of somatic intelligence that can't be rushed or borrowed. It must be earned through the practice of presence and attention. Our enteric nervous system, with its five hundred million neurons—more than in our spinal cord—serves as both sentinel and sage, a testament to the profound intelligence that resides within us, waiting to be heard and heeded.

As we journey into our Second Prime, our gut undergoes its own transformation, much like an experienced gardener adapting to changing seasons. Research shows that after age sixty, the diversity of our gut microbiome typically decreases by 10 to 15 percent, rather like losing some of our most skilled gardeners. The protective mucus layer in our gut also thins, making us more susceptible to inflammation and less resilient to dietary indiscretions that we might have shrugged off in our younger years.

Remember those legendary recovery powers after a night of debauchery in your twenties? The swift bounce back wasn't just youthful vigor. It was your gut microbiome working at peak efficiency. As we age, our digestive system becomes less forgiving, not out of spite, but because the intricate dance between our immune system and gut bacteria becomes more delicate. The production of essential compounds like short-chain fatty acids, which help maintain our gut barrier, naturally decreases with age. It's rather like our internal chemistry lab running on reduced hours.

But here's the fascinating bit. While aging inevitably affects our gut health, research suggests that many of these changes aren't simply the march of time, but rather the accumulation of lifestyle choices. Studies show that older adults who maintain diverse, plant-rich diets and regular physical activity often display gut microbiome profiles more similar to those decades younger. You can keep your microbiome fit and flourishing when you support its needs.

Have you ever noticed feeling a bit down after a weekend of indulging in high-fat foods and alcohol? It's not just the alcohol, a known depressant, that's to blame. The harmful gut microbes that thrive on an indulgent lifestyle of highly processed foods directly influence your mood and can leave you feeling exhausted, irritable, and blue. This phenomenon is all too common with the Standard American Diet—aptly abbreviated as SAD. Every time you eat, you're not just feeding yourself; you're feeding trillions of microorganisms that, in turn, produce metabolites that can cross the blood-brain barrier and influence your energy level, mood, cognition, motivation, and more.

Ah, the eternal battle with that chocolate chip cookie calling your name from the cupboard, just one or two. But before you blame your willpower (or lack thereof), let's consider the fascinating possibility that you're receiving a carefully organized message from billions of microscopic beings with their own agenda. Rather cheeky of them, isn't it?

With a high dose of self-compassion, it's nice to know that cravings for sugar or alcohol are often more than mere battles of will. These cravings are, in fact, the desperate cries of SOS sent by specific gut microbes that have adapted to thrive on sugary substances, producing signals that make us yearn for another bite or sip. The food industry has engineered highly processed foods to trigger these insane cravings. They call it the bliss point—though I dare say there's nothing particularly blissful about being manipulated by one's own microbes. These internal signals, once understood, become less like tyrannical demands and more like messages from a part of ourselves that needs attention and care. Understanding this biological dialogue transforms the narrative from one of willpower and shame to one of deeper self-awareness—a crucial shift as we navigate our Second Prime with growing wisdom.

The science behind this microbial manipulation is rather extraordinary. Certain bacteria, particularly species with fun names like *Prevotella* and *Bacteroides*, have developed sophisticated chemical signaling systems that interact directly with our vagus nerve, sending "feed me sugar!" telegrams to our brain. I think of the movie *Little Shop of Horrors* and the plant Audrey II singing to Seymour—a perfect metaphor for these microscopic manipulators who, like the carnivorous plant, have evolved their persuasive abilities over millions of years.

Think of it like they're banging on the pipes in an apartment to get your attention. These shrewd little organisms can even trigger the release of dopamine—our reward neurotransmitter—when we consume their preferred foods, creating a complex dance of craving and satisfaction that grows more intricate with each sugary morsel. It's rather like having millions of tiny addiction specialists working around the clock to influence our dietary choices, their ancient wisdom of survival sometimes at odds with our modern understanding of health. Yet understanding this internal chorus of voices gives us the power to respond rather than react, to listen with curiosity rather than surrender to their demands.

For some, like me, it only takes one or two sugary treats to kick off an intense craving for more, more, more. When I crave more sugar, I've become what one might call a puppet to these microscopic puppet masters. When fed their favored diet, these sugar-loving bacteria can double their population in a matter of hours, literally strengthening their voting power in the gut-brain congress. As we age, this microbial influence can become even more pronounced because our metabolism and insulin sensitivity naturally shifts. Think of insulin sensitivity as your body's ability to efficiently respond to sugar in your bloodstream. With age, this response can become less precise, making it all the more crucial to understand these internal dynamics.

The plot thickens when we consider that these sugar-craving microbes don't just influence our food choices; they can alter our taste receptors and reward pathways. It's diabolical! Research has shown that individuals with a higher proportion of these sugar-loving bacteria have up to 20 percent more active sweet taste receptors on their tongue. When you think about it, we're being reprogrammed from the inside out, a rather brilliant coup d'état.

But here's where it gets even more interesting. By understanding this cause and effect, we can turn the tables on our microscopic manipulators. When we make informed choices to starve these sugar-loving microbes, we simultaneously create conditions for their more beneficial cousins to thrive and replace them. These good bacteria, particularly species like *Akkermansia muciniphila* and various *Lactobacillus* strains found in fermented dairy, yogurt, and kefir, will help reduce inflammation and support metabolic health. They're the sort of tenants you want in your gut's neighborhood.

Your Second Prime is more than just about dieting to stay fit. It's about harnessing the power to replace harmful microbes with healthy, life-sustaining, joy-producing, disease-preventing ones. Think of it as a rather sophisticated form of biological diplomacy. We're not just fighting cravings; we're negotiating with an entire microscopic civilization to be able to live the life we envision. The more harmony you develop with your beneficial microbes, the more empowered you feel. It's like having trillions of supportive gladiators in your corner, each contributing to your resilience and vitality.

But here's the rub. This enhanced efficiency paradoxically occurs alongside a general decline in microbial diversity. Research shows that by age seventy, we typically lose about 25 percent of the bacterial species we had in our youth. But don't let this statistic worry you; we have a plan. This loss of diversity can make our internal ecosystem more vulnerable to disruption, rather like an economy overly dependent on a single industry.

The journey into our Second Prime brings distinct changes to our gut landscape, starting as early as forty. Our digestive enzyme production decreases by roughly 10 percent each decade.

The protective mucus layer in our gut thins significantly with age, with research in mice showing as much as an 80 percent reduction in thickness, making us more susceptible to irritation from foods we once enjoyed with abandon. Belly bloat, anyone? Studies show that after fifty, the beneficial *Bifidobacterium* species—our defenders against inflammation—typically decline by up to 30 percent. When we consider the modern everyday challenges and assaults our aging microbiome faces, it's a miracle that we are not all sick in the hospital with chronic illness. The average person over sixty takes four prescription medications daily, each potentially altering our microbial landscape. Common medications like proton pump inhibitors for acid reflux can reduce beneficial bacteria by up to 20 percent, while certain antibiotics can diminish our microbial diversity for up to two years after a single course.

This pharmaceutical influence on our gut health isn't a little disruption. It's an intense battle for survival on a microscopic level. Consider how many of us reach for an antacid without a second thought or accept multiple courses of antibiotics without considering probiotic supplementation. We've become rather casual about prescription medication, haven't we?

And speaking of modern habits that challenge our aging microbiome, let's consider three more rather inconvenient truths we often overlook. First, there's our casual relationship with NSAIDs—those seemingly innocent pain relievers we pop like after-dinner mints. Each tablet creates tiny tears in our gut lining, like taking sandpaper to delicate silk. It's quite cringeworthy when you think of it that way. Research suggests regular use can reduce beneficial bacteria by up to 50 percent. Mind-blowing when you consider the average person over fifty takes around two thousand of these tablets annually.

Then there's the matter of chronic dehydration, a silent

assassin of microbial health. As we age, our thirst signals become increasingly subtle, like a doorbell with failing batteries not ringing at all. By the time we feel thirsty, we're already significantly dehydrated. This parched environment makes it difficult for our beneficial bacteria to thrive, affecting everything from nutrient absorption to immune response.

And finally, there's the fiber gap, the modern dilemma. While our ancestors consumed upward of fifty grams of fiber daily, most of us manage barely fifteen. Our little residents need this crucial substrate to produce those beneficial short-chain fatty acids I mentioned earlier. Without adequate fiber, they're rather like craftsmen without their tools, like a construction site with workers just sitting around on the job, scrolling on their phones.

Throughout this book I highlight the importance of viewing ourselves as a unified whole, where the body, mind, and soul are deeply interconnected. However, we often fall into the habit of compartmentalizing, focusing too much on one aspect while neglecting the others. We sprint through our days, consuming pre-packaged convenience food while our inner pharmacy—that remarkable constellation of microorganisms—signals for something more authentic, more aligned with our true nature. Recent research has revealed intriguing data: When we're disconnected from our purpose, our gut microbiome literally changes its composition, influencing everything from our stress response to our cognitive clarity.

The science behind this vital connection is remarkable. Studies from the University of California have revealed that individuals with a powerful sense of purpose show up to 40 percent greater diversity in their gut microbiome compared to those feeling disconnected from their calling. This increased diversity translates to tangible health benefits, such as a 50 percent reduction in inflammatory markers, enhanced production of short-chain fatty acids that protect brain health, and significantly higher levels of neuro-transmitter precursors essential for emotional well-being.

Even more fascinating is how quickly our microbiome responds to changes in our sense of purpose and engagement. Research published in *The Journal of Positive Psychology* demonstrated that just two weeks of purposeful activity led to measurable changes in gut bacteria composition, with increases in beneficial species like *Lactobacillus* and *Bifidobacterium*—key players in mood regulation and immune function. These bacteria, in turn, produce compounds that enhance neuroplasticity and cognitive resilience, creating a positive feedback loop between purpose and brain health.

The metabolic conversation between our gut and our sense of purpose goes even deeper. When we engage in meaningful activities, our bodies show a 30 percent increase in the diversity of metabolites produced by gut bacteria. These metabolites, including specific short-chain fatty acids like butyrate (found in fiber-rich foods such as garlic, yogurt, and more), cross the blood-brain barrier and literally help rewrite our brain's emotional patterns. It's as if our microbiome responds to and reinforces our life's purpose through a complex chemical dialogue.

This connection becomes particularly crucial in our Second Prime. A longitudinal study following adults over sixty found that those maintaining strong purpose-driven activities showed remarkably different gut profiles compared to less engaged peers. The purpose-driven group maintained higher levels of anti-inflammatory species and demonstrated greater resilience against age-related decline in microbial diversity. Their gut bacteria produced 25 percent more compounds associated with cognitive protection and emotional well-being—a biological affirmation that living with purpose isn't only beneficial for our inner self, it's essential for the body.

Research has shown a 35 percent decrease in beneficial neurotransmitter precursors during periods of living inauthentically or leading unfulfilling lives. It's as if our inner pharmacy knows when we're not living authentically and sends chemical messages urging us toward our true path. The gut knows. You can try to ignore it, but as many of us intuit, the body tells the story. These signals become more pronounced with age, like an internal compass that's been calibrated by decades of experience. Studies of adults in their Second Prime reveal that this gut-wisdom often peaks in our sixties and seventies, perhaps nature's way of compensating for what we might lose in physical resilience with gains in intuitive intelligence.

When we are out of energetic alignment, suppress our inconvenient dreams, or stay in toxic relationships, we're not just squandering our full potential—we're actively working against our body's profound biological wisdom. The microbiome of individuals under chronic stress from life misalignment shows patterns eerily similar to those seen in accelerated aging. But here's the beautiful twist—research shows that it's never too late to course-correct. Our gut bacteria can begin shifting within days of making authentic choices, like stepping onto a new path or embarking on transformative travels.

Instead of settling, explore your passions and get lost in doing things you love. Your inconvenient dream is more than your purpose; it's an integral part of your gut health regimen. Think of it as a prescription for vitality, one that becomes more potent as we age. Each authentic choice, each step toward that dream you've kept tucked away, signals your microbiome to optimize for longevity and resilience rather than mere survival.

Perhaps this is why travel—that great leap into the unknown—speaks so profoundly to our spirit and internal ecosystem. When we venture beyond our familiar shores, we're not just crossing

geographical boundaries; we're answering an ancient call that resonates through every cell of our being. The sheer joy of discovery,
that delicious anticipation of what lies around the next corner, is
medicine for our microbiome. Research shows that positive emotions trigger the release of beneficial compounds that nourish our
gut bacteria, creating a beautiful cycle where joy feeds health and
health feeds joy.

Here's a delightful twist in our microbiome story: Travel is a
brilliant strategy for enhancing our internal diversity. Studies show
that immersing ourselves in different food cultures can introduce
hundreds of novel, beneficial bacterial species to our gut ecosystem.
It's like hosting an international symposium in your microbiome,
each new destination bringing unique diplomats to the party, each
moment of joy creating a cascade of beneficial effects that ripple
through our entire internal ecosystem. Our microbial companions, it seems, are rather fond of adventure themselves, thriving
on novel experiences, varied foods, and the pure, unbridled joy
that travel brings to our lives.

Consider how the Hadza hunter-gatherers of Tanzania show
seasonal shifts in their gut microbiome as they move and change
their diets—a reminder that our ancestors' nomadic patterns may
have contributed to their robust internal ecosystems. When we
travel, especially when we embrace local cuisines and traditional
fermented foods, we're not just collecting memories but cultivating
a more diverse and resilient internal community. Our nomadic
history of searching for food and water also may have had a beneficial side effect supporting a biological imperative for maintaining
our microbial diversity. This is an approach to support your gut
in your Second Prime while supporting a growth mindset. It's a
supportive framework for your mind, body, and spirit as you age,
seek, experience, nurture, and grow.

Of course, there's a clever way to approach travel for optimal gut benefits. While jet lag and travel stress might temporarily disrupt our microbiome, the long-term benefits of increased diversity can be remarkable. It's about finding that sweet spot between adventure and nurture, between exploring new gastronomic territories and supporting our gut's ability to adapt and thrive.

The following factors play a significant role in shaping your microbiome, some of which we've discussed throughout this chapter, but listed here together for ease of reference. By understanding these key factors, you can make informed choices to nurture and maintain a healthy microbiome.

- **Diet and alcohol:** What you eat and drink profoundly impacts the diversity and composition of your gut microbiota. Diets rich in fiber, fruits, vegetables, and fermented foods help foster a healthy microbiome, while those high in sugar, fat, and processed foods can disrupt it.

- **Genetics:** Your genetic makeup influences the types of bacteria that thrive in your gut. Some individuals may naturally be predisposed to specific microbial profiles.

- **Environment:** Your surroundings, including where you live and your exposure to nature, pets, and animals, can shape your microbiome.

- **Birth Method:** Babies delivered vaginally are exposed to their mother's bacteria, which helps establish their microbiome, whereas cesarean births may result in a different microbial composition.

- **Breastfeeding vs. Formula Feeding:** Breastfeeding supports the development of a healthy microbiome by providing beneficial bacteria and crucial nutrients, while formula feeding can lead to a different bacterial profile.

- **Age:** Your microbiome evolves with you, changing at various stages of life—from infancy to old age—each marked by distinct microbial characteristics.

- **Stress:** Chronic stress can alter the gut microbiota, disrupting its balance and potentially leading to health issues.

- **Antibiotic Use:** Antibiotics disrupt the balance of gut bacteria by killing both harmful and beneficial microbes. Overuse or unnecessary use can lead to lasting alterations in the microbiome.

- **Medications and Drug Use:** Beyond antibiotics, medicines like proton pump inhibitors, NSAIDs, and antipsychotics can affect the microbiome, sometimes negatively.

- **Infections and Illnesses:** Gastrointestinal infections and other illnesses can temporarily or permanently disrupt the microbial balance in the gut.

- **Hygiene Practices:** Overly sterile environments and excessive reliance on sanitizers and antibiotics can limit exposure to beneficial microbes, reducing microbial diversity.

- **Travel:** Traveling to new environments and experiencing different diets can introduce new microbes to your gut, potentially altering its balance.

- **Sleep Patterns:** Poor or irregular sleep disrupts the microbiome, while consistent, quality sleep supports health and stability.

The rest of this chapter offers some specific information about how gut bacteria functions and practical applications that you can try to foster a supportive environment for a healthy and well-functioning microbiome in your Second Prime.

First, we'll look at food and timing. Like us, our microbial companions operate on precise circadian rhythms, with research showing distinct patterns of metabolic activity:

- Peak digestive enzyme production occurs between 10 AM and 2 PM, so it's advisable to schedule your largest meal in this timeframe.

- Nutrient absorption is 40 percent more efficient in the morning hours, which means it's useful to frontload protein consumption in the first half of the day. Another good tip for nutrient absorption is to aim for twenty to forty chews for each bite.

- Inflammatory markers rise by 25 percent when we eat late at night, so avoid eating within three hours of bedtime.

- Gut repair processes are most active between 11 PM and 6 AM. To help out your gut, allow for twelve to fourteen hours of overnight fasting.

Also relating to food is the idea of strategic supplementation. As enzyme production naturally decreases with age, consider boosting yours using the following steps:

- Take digestive enzymes with meals (especially lipase and protease).

- Seek out specific probiotic strains depending on what you'd like to support, such as *L. rhamnosus GG* for immune support or *B. longum* for cognitive function.

- Add prebiotics, like inulin and FOS, which trigger the growth of good bacteria.

As discussed, diversity in the microbiome is key. And while travel is a great way to do that, you can also up your diversity with different kinds of foods. Research from the American Gut Project reveals that people consuming thirty or more different plant foods weekly show 50 percent greater microbiome diversity than those consuming fewer than ten. Here's how to achieve this:

- Six different leafy greens weekly (kale, spinach, arugula)
- Four different cruciferous vegetables weekly (broccoli, cauliflower, Brussels sprouts)
- Three different fermented foods weekly (kimchi, sauerkraut, kefir)
- Two types of resistant starch weekly (cooled potatoes, green bananas)
- Three differently colored fruits daily
- Two tablespoons of mixed seeds daily

There are also environmental factors at play. Exposure to diverse environments can boost immune function within twenty-four hours, so it's a great idea to get out as much as you can, even if that means walking in a different park or neighborhood than you usually do. Nature exposure significantly impacts microbiome diversity, and walking in forests increases natural killer cell activity by 40 percent. If you don't have access to a forest, your backyard will do: thirty minutes of gardening can introduce over two hundred beneficial bacterial species. To take advantage of environmental bacteria, here are some practical steps you can try:

- Create a small herb garden (even windowsill pots count!).
- Practice earthing/grounding for ten minutes daily.

- Exercise outdoors when possible.
- Reduce excessive household sanitization.

Research shows that there is a clear stress-microbiome connection. Chronic stress can reduce beneficial bacteria by up to 30 percent. But you can combat this through the following steps:

- Vagus nerve stimulation (humming, gargling, deep breathing)
- Mindful eating practices (shown to improve digestion by 40 percent)
- Regular movement (even fifteen minutes of post-meal walking helps)
- Stress-reduction techniques tied to mealtimes

Challenge: Power Up Your Microbiome in Thirty Days

Remember, this journey isn't about perfection. It's about partnership with the remarkable universe within. Each small choice, whether it's introducing a new fermented food or taking that gentle evening walk, becomes part of a larger dialogue with your internal wisdom. The transformative power lies not in dramatic overhauls but in these daily acts of conscious attention.

Your microbiome awaits your care, not with demands for immediate mastery, but with an invitation to gradual, profound partnership. Sometimes the most significant changes begin with something as simple as a spoonful of sauerkraut or a mindful walk under the evening sky. Here is a thirty-day challenge to jumpstart better gut health.

Week 1: Awaken the Ancient Wisdom

Like those resilient archaea we discussed, your microbiome carries profound adaptive wisdom. This week, begin listening to its subtle language:

- Choose one meal a day to eat without distractions, honoring the gut-brain dialogue we explored.
- Take three deep breaths before meals, activating your vagus nerve's calming influence.
- Begin with one gentle fermented food, perhaps a few spoonfuls of plain yogurt or a sip of kombucha in the afternoon.
- After dinner, embrace a ten-minute ceremonial walk, a gentle movement that research shows can enhance digestion by up to 17 percent.

Week 2: Cozy Up to Your Internal Ecosystem

Memory is a curious landscape, especially when it comes to our relationship with nourishment. This week, deepen your exploration.

- Expand your fermented food repertoire by adding raw sauerkraut (start with one tablespoon) to your lunch, or experiment with milk kefir in your morning routine. Introduce miso soup or kimchi. Remember to start slowly—these are potent allies that deserve respect.
- Practice the art of the post-meal pause. Take a leisurely ten- to fifteen-minute walk after your largest meal, allowing your body to find that delicate balance between movement and digestion.

- Create space between dinner and sleep (aim for three hours) to honor your microbiome's natural rhythms.

Week 3: Embrace Purpose Through Partnership

Our inconvenient dreams aren't obstacles but invitations to deeper nourishment. This week focusses on that profound connection.

- Notice which fermented foods resonate most with your system (perhaps the tang of water kefir or the umami of traditional pickled vegetables).
- Align your movement patterns with your body's wisdom— gentle walks after meals rather than vigorous exercise.
- Add more advanced fermented options if ready.
- Create rituals that honor both movement and rest (perhaps a morning stretch followed by a mindful breakfast).

Week 4: Integration and Evolution

Like the intricate connection between gut and brain that we explored, this week weaves together all you've discovered.

- Establish your personal rhythm of fermented foods. Which ones bring vitality? Which times of day feel most nourishing?
- Fine-tune your movement patterns. Try a morning stretch, post-meal walk, and evening unwinding.
- Create your sustainable practice of post-meal movement, finding that sweet spot between activity and rest.
- Honor your internal ecosystem's wisdom in choosing foods and movement that resonate deeply.

Glimmers and Wisdom: The Gift of Enhanced Joy!

Life has a fascinating way of revealing its most profound gifts precisely when we're ready to receive them. As we journey through our Second Prime, that magical phase where wisdom meets vitality, we discover an unexpected superpower: the ability to find extraordinary joy in life's ordinary moments. By reading this book, you've already made the empowering choice to embrace the goodness and beauty surrounding you and approach your Second Prime with attention and intention. This conscious decision will enrich each day with your wealth of experience, seamlessly intertwining it with newfound possibilities.

That stunning, awe-inspiring sunset that you would have barely noticed twenty years ago stops you in your tracks when viewed with a mind seeking to find the good, the beautiful, and the remarkable that is present all around us. The laughter of children playing in the distance resonates differently, carrying echoes of your own joy across decades. This isn't just nostalgia; it's the Second Prime advantage, where our seasoned perspective transforms fleeting moments into profound experiences.

I am delighted to share a concept that brought me a spark of joy—learning about *glimmers*, a term coined by pioneering social worker Dr. Deb Dana. A glimmer is more than just a delightful moment; it's a gentle awakening of the nervous system, a whispered reminder that amid life's complexities, beauty and safety still exist in abundance. Unlike the jarring nature of triggers that set off our fight-or-flight response, glimmers are those subtle instances when our body remembers its capacity for peace, wonder, and connection. When a glimmer washes over us, something extraordinary happens. A flood of positive neurochemicals and warm emotions infuses our entire being. Imagine your nervous system as a constellation of stars, each point of light representing a neural pathway. When a glimmer arrives—perhaps that first sip of perfectly brewed coffee or the sound of a loved one's laughter—it ignites a cascade of well-being.

In these precious moments, your body becomes a biochemical orchestra of joy. Your hypothalamus—the conductor of this biological symphony—signals dopamine release. This pleasure neurotransmitter creates that delicious surge of warmth in your chest. Simultaneously, oxytocin begins to flow, creating that sense of connection and contentment that makes you feel at one with the world. Serotonin levels rise, painting your world in brighter hues, while endorphins create that subtle euphoria that makes you want to pause and savor the moment.

In this cheer-filled chapter, we'll delve into the enchanting world of glimmers. Yes, they are real! And in our Second Prime we're uniquely positioned to harness their power. These micro-moments of joy aren't just pleasant diversions. They're potent catalysts for well-being, backed by fascinating research from the Harvard Study of Adult Development showing that those who cultivate the ability to savor positive experiences demonstrate markedly better health outcomes and greater life satisfaction.

Glimmers are nature's subtle rebellion against life's shadows. They are tiny bursts of joy that dance through our consciousness like fireflies on a summer evening. These moments aren't just poetic interludes; they're powerful neurological events that release a cascade of positive neurotransmitters, including dopamine and serotonin, creating a biological scaffold of safety. While our ancestors needed Keep Calm and Carry On to weather literal storms and war, I propose a gentler wisdom for our modern trials—Keep

Calm and Glimmer On!

My most cherished glimmer arrived with delightful unexpect-
edness, as the best ones often do. Standing outside a Southern
California dry cleaner's—that temple of mundane errands—I
found myself absentmindedly studying the building's stucco wall,
its multidimensional color and texture a topographical map of
countless tiny peaks and valleys. Like thousands of its architectural
siblings dotting the landscape, it featured the requisite built-in
planter, hosting a drowsy congregation of impatiens nodding in
the summer heat. I gave it the contents of my water bottle.

Then I saw them—a civilization in miniature. Two precise
lines of ants, moving with the choreographed precision of a tiny
metropolis at rush hour. Each ant, barely larger than a punctuation
mark on the page of this book, participated in an elaborate ritual of
acknowledgment as they passed their colleagues, touching anten-
nae in what I couldn't help but interpret as micro-namastes. Some
carried fragments of their world—pebbles and plant matter that,
relative to their size, would make Olympic weightlifters jealous.
Others seemed to serve as traffic directors, information brokers, or
perhaps the ant equivalent of workplace social coordinators.

What captivated me wasn't just their industry but their
interconnectedness. In an age where human society often feels
increasingly fragmented, these tiny beings demonstrated an ancient wisdom about the power of collective purpose. Each brief
antenna touch represented millions of years of evolutionary choreography, a reminder that communication—even at its most
basic—is the thread that weaves individual existence into commu-
nal success.

My impromptu meditation on ant society ended, but the
wonder lingered. I found myself diving into ant research with the
enthusiasm of a child discovering dinosaurs for the first time. This,
I realized, is the true magic of glimmers. They're not just moments

of joy, but portals to deeper curiosity and connection. In an era where we're often urged to think bigger, my most profound insight came from thinking smaller, from recognizing that even the most seemingly insignificant moments can open windows to wonder in our Second Prime.

This glimmer struck such a deep chord because it embodied what developmental psychologists call mature fascination—the ability to find profound meaning in simple observations that develops as we age. It reminded me that wisdom isn't just about accumulating knowledge but about maintaining the capacity to be wonderstruck by the ordinary. What is more ordinary than a row of ants? In our Second Prime, we're uniquely positioned to appreciate these moments, having developed crystallized intelligence—the ability to connect new observations with a lifetime of accumulated understanding.

The science behind these magical moments is as fascinating as the experience itself. Dana's groundbreaking work has been further validated by a 2023 study in *The Journal of Positive Psychology*, revealing that individuals who actively practiced glimmer awareness experienced a profound transformation—a 47 percent increase in reported daily life satisfaction and a remarkable 38 percent reduction in stress hormone levels.

But here's where the journey becomes even more extraordinary for those of us in our Second Prime. We've developed emotional granularity; a sophisticated ability to identify and savor the subtle variations in positive experiences. Think of it as developing a connoisseur's palate for joy, where each moment carries its own unique flavor and resonance.

Glimmer awareness isn't merely about noticing lovely moments. It's an intentional practice of discovering and collecting tiny bursts of wonder that punctuate our daily lives. It might be the way morning light catches dewdrops on a spider's web, the familiar creak of your favorite chair, or the particular sound of a loved one's laughter. These micro-moments of delight serve as natural antidotes to our brain's inherent negativity bias, an evolutionary holdover that's become increasingly unnecessary in our modern world.

Research from the University of California's Greater Good Science Center has shown that individuals who cultivate glimmer awareness demonstrate enhanced neuroplasticity—the brain's ability to form new neural pathways. This is particularly significant for those of us in our Second Prime, as it challenges the outdated notion that our capacity for joy and wonder diminishes with age. Instead, we're discovering that our accumulated life experience provides a richer context for appreciating these moments, like expert artists who have spent decades learning to see the subtle interplay of light and shadow.

The practice of glimmer awareness follows a beautiful paradox. The more we train ourselves to notice these moments, the more abundant they become. It's as if we're tuning our internal radio to a frequency of joy that's been broadcasting all along. Neuroscientists have observed that this practice strengthens the prefrontal cortex's positive attention networks, making it easier to spot and savor these moments of micro-joy over time.

For those beginning this practice, start with anchored awareness—choosing specific daily activities as prompts for noticing glimmers. Perhaps it's your morning coffee ritual, the evening walk with your dog, or the moment you first step outside each day. These anchors become reliable opportunities to practice spotting the extraordinary within the ordinary, training our minds to become skilled hunters of joy rather than collectors of worry.

The beauty of developing glimmer awareness in our Second Prime lies in its cumulative effect. Like compound interest for the soul, each noticed moment builds upon the last, gradually transforming our default perspective from one of scarcity to one of abundance. We begin to see that age hasn't diminished our capacity for wonder—it's enhanced it, giving us a deeper appreciation for life's subtle symphonies.

One of my favorite glimmers is simply the word *glimmer* itself; it's as though the word carries its own spark of enchantment. When I think of it, I feel a joyful charge bloom in my chest, like stars awakening at twilight. It conjures images of glitter catching light, of all things magical, fresh, and luminously, sparkly, pretty and, well, . . . glittery! It transports me back to that pure, boundless wonder I felt when I believed in fairies dancing through garden shadows and elves leaving tiny footprints in morning dew. It reminds me of childhood treasures; those intricate panoramic sugared easter eggs that held entire worlds of possibility behind their delicate sugar-crystal windows.

I can actively fetch that feeling of joy and giddiness by simply whispering "glimmer" to myself. Give it a try! It's like uncorking a bottle of pure delight, releasing bubbles of joy that fizz through your consciousness. I imagine my cells as tiny prisms, each one illuminating in sequence until my entire being glows with remembered magic. This isn't just whimsy; it's a conscious choice to reawaken that childlike ability to see wonder in everything, now enriched by our Second Prime wisdom that recognizes just how precious such moments truly are.

Here's where the magic of our Second Prime truly shines. Our mature nervous systems have developed positive resonance circuits. Like a well-tuned instrument, our bodies have learned to amplify and sustain these moments of joy. The rush you feel isn't just a fleeting sensation; it's your body's wisdom at work, having learned over decades to recognize and maximize these precious moments of pure delight.

When you actively recall a glimmer, as with your enchanting association with the word itself, you're not just remembering; you're reactivating these neural networks. Your anterior cingulate cortex—the brain region responsible for emotional awareness—lights up like a sunrise. Your amygdala—usually known for processing fear and scanning for danger—becomes a sanctuary for positive emotional memories. This is why the feeling can seem to ripple through your entire body. Because, in a very real sense *it does*!

This complex biological activity of well-being isn't just beautiful. It's transformative. Each glimmering moment strengthens these positive neural pathways, making finding and savoring future moments of joy easier. It's as though we're creating a constellation map of happiness, each glimmer adding another bright point to guide us toward well-being.

These micro-joys are not just fleeting moments but gentle reminders that life is about more than mere survival—it's about thriving. And in our Second Prime, we're not just collecting happy moments; we're actively creating a legacy of joy that ripples outward, touching the lives of those around us. This is where the true magic of Second Prime glimmers lies—in their ability to transform our experience and create a contagious atmosphere of possibility and delight benefiting everyone in our orbit. Glimmers are gifts we can notice and give to each other.

Step into your local coffee shop on any given morning and there's your barista, already crafting your perfectly customized drink before you speak. While this thoughtful gesture brightens anyone's day, fascinating research from the Stanford Center on Longevity reveals how our brain's processing of such moments evolves as we age.

Picture a beloved symphony playing. Both a twenty-five-year-old and a fifty-five-year-old might be equally moved by the music. However, brain imaging studies show our mature minds have developed additional neural pathways that weave these experiences into more complex layers of meaning. The anterior cingulate cortex forms stronger connections with memory centers as we age, creating enhanced pattern recognition for social connection.

This biological evolution transforms our morning coffee ritual into something deeper in our Second Prime. These brief but genuine interactions contribute to cumulative positive effects, building cognitive resilience and emotional equilibrium over time. It's as if our brains have developed a more sophisticated emotional palette capable of detecting subtle notes of connection in everyday moments.

Through decades of research at Stanford University, Dr. Laura Carstensen's groundbreaking socioemotional selectivity theory reveals something remarkable: Our maturing brains don't simply change, they evolve to enhance our capacity for joy and connection. This isn't about diminishing younger people's experiences. Rather, it's about recognizing how our neural architecture continues to develop in ways that deepen our appreciation for life's quiet moments of beauty.

Watch a butterfly alight on a nearby flower, wings catching sunlight. The same scene captivates viewers of any age, but neuroscience shows our seasoned brains have developed enhanced perceptual discrimination—a refined ability to notice and savor life's subtle magnificence. This discovery aligns perfectly with our growing understanding of the aging brain's remarkable plasticity and wisdom.

Complementing this understanding, a landmark study from the University of Michigan's Institute for Social Research tracked adults over three decades, unveiling the neural architecture of this enhancement. Following participants through their journey into Second Prime, researchers discovered heightened activity in the anterior cingulate cortex during positive micro-moments. Think of it as though our brains have spent decades fine-tuning their ability to detect and amplify life's subtle symphonies of joy.

Together, this research paints a magnificent picture of our

Second Prime potential. We're not just aging, we're evolving, our neural pathways becoming ever more attuned to life's glimmers of beauty and meaning.

Think of it as nature's magnificent compensation. While our younger selves might have processed more information more quickly, our Second Prime brains have evolved to process experiences more deeply. A 2022 study in the *Journal of Neuroscience* showed that adults in their Second Prime demonstrated a 34 percent increase in activity in the brain's pleasure centers when observing natural beauty compared to their younger counterparts. We're not just seeing the butterfly; we're experiencing it throughout our body, with our entire lifetime of accumulated wonder.

This enhanced awareness isn't limited to visual beauty. The same neural networks that help us notice the butterfly's dance also attune us to the rhythm of conversation, the subtle shift in a loved one's expression, and the perfect timing of a kind word. We've developed what researchers call *emotional expertise*—a sophisticated ability to recognize and appreciate life's meaningful moments that tends to improve as we age.

Dr. Barbara Fredrickson's research on micro-moments of positivity resonance adds another fascinating layer. Her studies show that these brief encounters with beauty—the wonders of nature or a flash of a stranger's genuine smile—trigger a cascade of beneficial neurochemicals.

When was the last time you stood in pure awe, your sense of self momentarily dissolved in the face of something greater? Science shows us that experiencing awe, big or small—whether gazing at the stars, standing before nature's grandeur, listening to music, enjoying a live performance, or marveling at art—literally expands our perspective and rewires our neural pathways. Each moment of astonishment reaches beyond happy diversions. They're powerful reset buttons for our nervous system, shifting us from a stress response to a state of profound appreciation and peace.

Your Second Prime brings a unique advantage to this experience. The sophisticated neural networks you've developed over decades allow you to perceive and process these moments with unprecedented depth. Research in positive psychology reveals that routinely experiencing such optimistic emotions doesn't just improve our mental state. It enhances physical health, reduces inflammatory stress responses, and can extend our lifespan.

Think of cultivating glimmers as training your brain's spotlight of attention. Instead of automatically scanning for problems (a primitive survival mechanism), you're teaching your mind to notice the shimmering possibilities that surround you. This isn't just positive thinking. It's a conscious rewiring of your neural pathways toward resilience and joy.

Challenge: Glimmer Hunting

In our Second Prime, we have a unique opportunity to transform our daily experience through intentional awareness and practiced joy. These challenges aren't mere activities; they're invitations to rediscover the world through our evolved capacity for wonder. In addition, these challenges aren't about adding more tasks to your day. They're about awakening to the extraordinary possibilities that already exist within ordinary moments. Your Second Prime has gifted you with the neural refinement to appreciate life's subtle beauties and the wisdom to understand their true value. Let each day become an adventure in glimmer-hunting, knowing that every moment of joy you discover, and share creates ripples of positive change in the world around you.

Choose one or two that resonate deeply with you, allowing them to become portals to a more enriched existence.

- **Morning Gratitude Ritual:** Begin each day by savoring three moments of gratitude, but with a Second Prime twist. Instead of simply listing them, explore *why* they matter to you now in ways they might not have in your younger years. Let your seasoned perspective illuminate the deeper significance of what you once might have taken for granted.

- **Nature's Whispers:** Take mindful walks where your sole purpose is discovering glimmers in nature's subtle displays. Notice how differently you perceive these moments now. How a dewdrop catching morning light might hold your attention in ways it never could before. Your mature nervous system is uniquely attuned to appreciate these quiet symphonies of beauty.

- **Legacy of Kindness:** Transform ordinary interactions into extraordinary moments of connection. When the barista remembers your order, pause to deeply appreciate this moment of human connection. Share a story with a junior colleague, offering the kind of perspective that only comes with time. Each interaction becomes an opportunity to weave warmth into the fabric of someone else's day.

- **Creative Awakening:** Engage in activities that marry joy with growth. Learn to paint, write, or play music. Your Second Prime brain brings patience and perspective to the learning process, allowing you to find pleasure in the journey rather than rushing toward mastery.

- **Sunset Meditation:** End your day with conscious reflection. Watch the sky's transformation, allowing each color shift to remind you of your own beautiful evolution. Use this time to collect the day's glimmers, storing them like precious gems in your memory.

- **Connection Chronicles:** Reach out to someone who matters, not with a quick text, but with the kind of unhurried conversation that allows wisdom to surface naturally. Share memories, but more importantly, create new ones enriched by your Second Prime perspective.

- **Laughter Legacy:** Seek out what makes you laugh deeply and freely. Whether it's watching comedy, sharing jokes with friends, or simply finding humor in life's quirks, remember that joy shared is joy multiplied. Your laughter now carries the warmth of wisdom, making it even more infectious.

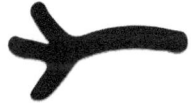

Conclusion: Purpose, Power, and Possibility

Questions shape our reality more profoundly than answers ever could. As we stand at what appears to be the close of our exploration, we find ourselves not at an ending but at the threshold of something far more remarkable—*your* Second Prime journey. Like the Seattle brunch where possibility first sparked into being for me, we return to the beginning with a fresh and knowledgeable perspective, a broader understanding—about ourselves, our society, our biology, our choices, and most importantly, our power to reshape how aging is understood and experienced.

Remember how a simple gathering of friends over Bloody Marys was a moment when ideas sparked and gave enough oxygen to smolder and catch fire? Where the possibilities and dreams we dared to call inconvenient first rooted in my mind as an effortless way to dream big without constraint? We've come back to that same place of infinite potential, but this time, we arrive transformed, armed not just with wisdom and science but with a profound understanding that the quality of our questions shapes the quality of our lives.

The research confirms what the slightly boozy brunch conversation intuited: Individuals who maintain strong social ties while pursuing meaningful goals experience up to a 50 percent reduction in mortality risk. But this statistic tells only part of the story. Each component we've explored—purpose, meaningful relationships, movement, mindfulness—compounds like interest, creating a remarkable return on investment for our future selves. Our journey together has revealed something extraordinary. This irreverent query that first started our exploration has led us to deeper waters, to questions that only life experience could help us formulate. Each chapter has peeled back another layer of possibility, showing us that when we change the questions we ask about aging, we transform how we experience it.

The science speaks clearly: Purpose-driven living adds years to your life—outperforming even quitting smoking or starting exercise. But the real story? Men and women navigate this aging landscape with different maps. Women's social connections aren't just pleasant—they're survival tools, creating measurable differences in longevity outcomes.

Our biological advantages in aging aren't guarantees for women—they're opportunities and invitations requiring cultivation. Our tendency toward deeper social networks and willingness to share vulnerabilities creates protective barriers against the isolation men often struggle to build. Men typically maintain fewer close relationships and share less emotional content within them—not because they prefer isolation but because they've been taught different relational languages altogether.

Your Second Prime isn't about fighting against your biology—it's about working with it intelligently. Understanding these patterns of biological sex empowers you to write your longevity story, regardless of which side you started from.

When we combine purposeful living with strong social connections, our bodies respond at the cellular level. Our telomeres (those protective caps on our DNA) actually lengthen, while our emotional intelligence (that capacity to understand and navigate complex feelings) deepens with each passing year. This isn't just about preserving youth; it's about evolving into something more sophisticated, nuanced, and powerful than our younger selves could imagine. And it all begins with taking control of our narrative and embracing the power of community.

In today's excessively dynamic world, it can be easy to get caught up in the never-ending cycle of work, sleep, and repeat. Like an ancient wisdom waiting to be rediscovered, our research into the mind-body connection revealed layers of possibility we're only beginning to understand. Those who maintain diverse gut bacteria through mindful eating and stress management show 40 percent lower inflammation markers and significantly better cognitive function. But beyond these numbers lies a more profound truth; our capacity for joy expands with time.

Those glimmers we explored—those micro-moments when joy lights up our nervous system—become richer and more meaningful in our Second Prime. Our mature brains have developed enhanced perceptual discrimination, allowing us to savor life's subtle magnificence with unprecedented depth. A shared laugh with an old friend, the warmth of morning sunlight, the satisfaction of mentoring someone through a challenge—these aren't just pleasant moments but powerful catalysts for well-being.

Consider how these elements build upon each other. Regular meditation reduces biological age markers, while spiritual practices lower the risk of depression and anxiety. When we add meaningful work or volunteering, cognitive function improves and the risk of dementia drops. This isn't just about preventing decline—it's about accessing new levels of vitality and connectedness that only become possible with the wisdom of years.

The power of this transformation reveals itself not through statistics but through the careful observation of lives unfolding with purpose. Each choice to remain engaged—whether through work, creativity, or service—creates ripples that extend far beyond ourselves. Those who maintain economic engagement while pursuing their purpose are healthier and live longer, supporting that contribution isn't simply good for society; it's essential for our own well-being.

Through each challenge in this book, you've discovered something powerful about autonomy and agency—the ability to shape your journey isn't diminished by time but enhanced by experience. When we reclaim authorship of our story and choose growth over comfort and purpose over passive existence, we improve our lives and help rewrite society's narrative about what's possible in our later years.

The transformation we seek doesn't require grandiose gestures. It grows from small, conscious choices—a mindful meal shared with friends, a moment to truly listen to your inner wisdom, a step toward that inconvenient dream that wouldn't stay quiet. Each choice creates a cascade of benefits, strengthening neural pathways, reducing stress hormones, and expanding our capacity for joy and resilience in measurable ways.

Think of how differently we understand power now compared to our younger years. Where once we might have sought control through force of will or external validation, we've discovered a more nuanced form of agency—one that flows from alignment with our deepest values and truths. This isn't the brash confidence of youth but something far more priceless: the quiet certainty that comes from knowing who we are and what we stand for.

Consider the impact when one of us chooses to pursue a new venture at sixty or speaks about aging with pride instead of an apology or demonstrates through action that our Second Prime can be our most vital chapter. We become living permission slips for others to reimagine their own futures. These aren't just individual choices. They're acts of revolution against a culture that has too often equated aging with decline.

So, does aging suck, or do we suck at aging? Our journey has revealed that we've been asking the wrong question entirely. Or rather, we've been asking a low-quality question and getting precisely the low-quality experience to match. When we ask "Does aging suck?" we've already framed aging as potentially negative and ourselves as passive recipients. But the subtle shift to "Do we suck at aging?" puts the responsibility and opportunity squarely in our hands. This isn't mere wordplay—it's a fundamental reorientation of our relationship with time.

Aging itself is neutral, but the meaning we assign to it shapes our experience. How we choose to grow, contribute, and live fully in each moment matters. The science is strong, and the data is incredibly positive: Those who approach their Second Prime with intention—nurturing purpose, maintaining vibrant connections, and engaging actively with life—don't merely exist through additional years. They flourish in dimensions our youth-obsessed culture hasn't yet comprehended.

This shift in questioning transforms everything. When we stop asking how to reverse aging and start asking how to age brilliantly, we step into our power. The quality of our questions determines the quality of our lives.

Your role in this revolution is both simple and profound:

- Challenge limiting beliefs about aging wherever you encounter them.
- Create spaces that celebrate wisdom and experience.
- Build bridges between generations through authentic relationships.
- Share your accumulated wisdom while remaining open to learning.
- Reimagine work and contribution for longer lifespans.
- Support age-inclusive businesses and initiatives.
- Maintain curiosity and openness to growth.
- Share your unique gifts with the world.

Imagine meeting your future self, the one who stands ten, twenty years ahead on this path. Feel the quiet gratitude in their eyes for every small choice you're making today. See how their presence carries the accumulated power of purposeful living and how their energy radiates the vitality that comes from aligning with their most profound truth. With each step you take today— each time you choose to reach out to a friend, choose purpose over comfort and growth over stagnation—you're crafting a gift not just for your future self but for future generations.

The story of aging is being rewritten, and you hold the pen. But this isn't just your story; it's a chapter in humanity's greater narrative. Every time you embrace your Second Prime with intention and joy, you create ripples that touch countless lives. Each person who witnesses your transformation sees you pursuing your inconvenient dream with courage and recognizes the power of purposeful aging through your example. Then, they too become part of this meaningful revolution.

This is how cultural change happens. Not through grand gestures alone but through thousands of individual choices to live differently, to age consciously, and to embrace the full spectrum of human potential at every stage of life.

Together, let's create a world where the Second Prime isn't just a concept. It's a celebration of human potential fully realized; it's a societal assumption for the greater good—you can have as many Primes as you choose to create. The revolution of aging awaits, and it begins with you. And now, at the close of our exploration, the most critical question remains: What will you do with this one wild and precious Second Prime and beyond?

References

Chapter 1: Time Crimes: A Not-So-Pretty History of Our Aging Attitudes

Age Discrimination in Employment Act (ADEA) of 1967, 29 U.S.C. § 621–634.

Atkinson, H. H., et al. (2007). "Cognitive function, gait speed decline, and comorbidities: The health, aging and body composition study." *The Journals of Gerontology Series A: Biological Sciences and Medical Sciences*, 62(8), 844–850. doi.org/10.1093/gerona/62.8.844.

Bellingtier, J. A., & Neupert, S. D. (2018). "Negative aging attitudes predict greater reactivity to daily stressors in older adults." *The Journals of Gerontology: Series B*, 73(7), 1155–1159. doi.org/10.1093/geronb/gbw086.

Gagnon, C., Olmand, et al. (2022). "Videoconference version of the Montreal Cognitive Assessment: Normative data for Quebec-French people aged 50 years and older." *Aging Clinical and Experimental Research*, 34(7), 1627–1633. doi.org/10.1007/s40520-022-02092-1.

Kornadt, A. E., Siebert, J. S., & Wahl, H. W. (2019). "The interplay of personality and attitudes toward own aging across two decades of later life." *The Journals of Gerontology: Series B*, 74(5), 59–67. doi.org/10.1371/journal.pone.0223622.

Levy, B. R. (2003). "Mind matters: Cognitive and physical effects of aging self-stereotypes." *The Journals of Gerontology Series B: Psychological Sciences and Social Sciences*, 58(4), P203–P211. doi.org/10.1093/geronb/58.4.P203.

Levy, B.R., et al. (2016). "A culture-brain link: Negative age stereotypes predict Alzheimer's disease biomarkers." *Psychology and Aging*, 31(1), 82–88. doi.org/10.1037/pag0000062.

Levy, B. R., & Myers, L. M. (2004). "Preventive health behaviors influenced by self-perceptions of aging." *Preventive Medicine*, 39(3), 625–629. doi.org/10.1016/j.ypmed.2004.02.029.

Levy, B. R., Slade, M. D., Kunkel, S. R., & Kasl, S. V. (2002). "Longevity increased by positive self-perceptions of aging." *Journal of Personality and Social Psychology*, 83(2), 261–270. doi.org/10.1037/0022-3514.83.2.261.

Löckenhoff, C. E., et al. (2009). "Perceptions of aging across 26 cultures and their culture-level associates." *Psychology and Aging*, 24(4), 941–954. doi.org/10.1037/a0016901.

National Institute on Aging. (2024). "Cognitive health and older adults." U.S. Department of Health & Human Services. nia.nih.gov/health/brain-health/cognitive-health-and-older-adults.

O'Brien, E. L., & Sharifian, N. (2020). "Managing expectations: How stress, social support, and aging attitudes affect awareness of age-related changes." *Journal of Social and Personal Relationships*, 37(3), 986–1007. doi.org/10.1177/0265407519883009.

Park, M. S., Badham, S., Vizcaino-Vickers, S., & Fino, E. (2024). "Exploring older adults' subjective views on aging positively: Development and validation of the positive aging scale." *The Gerontologist*, 64(9), 1–10. doi.org/10.1093/geront/gnae088.

Piazza, J. R., et al. (2013). "Affective reactivity to daily stressors and long-term risk of reporting a chronic physical health condition." *Annals of Behavioral Medicine*, 45(1), 110–120. doi.org/10.1007/s12160-012-9423-0.

Rickard, N., et al. (2016). "Development of a mobile phone app to support self-monitoring of emotional well-being: A mental health digital innovation." *JMIR Mental Health*, 3(4), e49. doi.org/10.2196/mental.6202.

Sackett, P. R., Shewach, O. R., & Keiser, H. N. (2017). "Survey on attitudes toward aging." *Journal of Applied Psychology*, 102(10), 1409–1426. doi.org/10.1037/apl0000236.

Sargent-Cox, K. A., Anstey, K. J., & Luszcz, M. A. (2012). "The relationship between change in self-perceptions of aging and physical functioning in older adults." *Psychology and Aging*, 27(3), 750–760. doi.org/10.1037/a0027578.

Sindi, S., Juster, R. P., et al. (2012). "Depressive symptoms, cortisol, and cognition during human aging: The role of negative aging perceptions." *Stress*, 15(2), 130–137. doi.org/10.3109/10253890.2011.599047

Wurm, S., et al. (2017). "How do views on aging affect health outcomes in adulthood and late life? Explanations for an established connection." *Developmental Review*, 46, 27–43. doi.org/10.1016/j.dr.2017.08.002.

Wurm, S., Tomasik, M. J., & Tesch-Römer, C. (2010). "On the importance of a positive view on ageing for physical exercise among middle-aged and older adults: Cross-sectional and longitudinal findings." *Psychology & Health*, 25(1), 25–42. doi.org/10.1080/08870440802311314.

Chapter 2: Inconvenient Dreams: The Messengers We Try to Ignore

Boyle, P. A., et al. (2017). "Purpose in life and risk of mild cognitive impairment and progression to dementia: the rush memory and aging project." Archives of *General Psychiatry*, Rush Alzheimer's Disease Center.

Conley, C. (2018). *Wisdom at Work: The Making of a Modern Elder*. Currency Publishing.

Kim, E. S., et al. (2020). "Sense of purpose in life and five health behaviors in older adults." *Preventive Medicine, 139*: 106172.

Chapter 3: Beyond the Map: When Purpose Becomes Your North Star

Blanchflower, D. G., & Oswald, A. J. (2008). "Is well-being U-shaped over the life cycle?" *Social Science & Medicine, 66*(8): 1733–1749.

Carstensen, L. L., & DeLiema, M. (2018). "The positivity effect: A negativity bias in youth fades with age." *Current Opinion in Behavioral Sciences, 19*: 7–12.

Dweck, C. S. (2006). *Mindset: The New Psychology of Success*. Random House.

Levinson, D. J. (1978). *The Seasons of a Man's Life*. Ballantine Books.

Rauch, J. (2018). *The Happiness Curve: Why Life Gets Better After 50*. Thomas Dunne Books.

Schultz, W. (2016). "Dopamine reward prediction error coding." *Dialogues in Clinical Neuroscience, 18*(1): 23–32. doi.org/10.31887/DCNS.2016.18.1/wschultz.

Steger, M. F., et al. (2009). "Meaning in life across the life span: Levels and correlates of meaning in life from emerging adulthood to older adulthood." *The Journal of Positive Psychology, 4*(1): 43–52. psycnet.apa.org/doi/10.1080/17439760802303127.

Waxman, B. (2016). *The Middlescence Manifesto: Igniting the Passion of Midlife*. Self-published.

Chapter 4: The Midlife "Crisis": And Why It Is Really an Invitation

Carstensen, L. L. (2006). "The Influence of a Sense of Time on Human Development." *Science, 312*(5782): 1913–1915. doi.org/10.1126/science.1127488.

Conley, C. (2018). *Wisdom at Work: The Making of a Modern Elder*. Currency Publishing.

Jaques, E. (1965). "Death and the Mid-life Crisis." *International Journal of Psychoanalysis, 46*: 502–514.

Lachman, M. E. (2015). "Mind the gap in the middle: A call to study midlife." *Research in Human Development, 12*(3–4): 327–334. doi.org/10.1080/15427609.2015.1068048.

Park, D. C., & Reuter-Lorenz, P. (2009). "The adaptive brain: Aging and neurocognitive scaffolding." *Annual Review of Psychology, 60*: 173–196. pmc.ncbi.nlm.nih.gov/articles/PMC3359129.

Ryff, C. D. (2014). "Psychological well-being revisited: Advances in the science and practice of eudaimonia." *Psychotherapy and Psychosomatics, 83*(1): 10–28. pubmed.ncbi.nlm.nih.gov/24281296.

Chapter 5: The Future You: An Inside Job

Cirillo, F. (2006). *The Pomodoro Technique: The Acclaimed Time-Management System That Has Transformed How We Work*. Currency Publishing.

Clear, J. (2018). *Atomic Habits: An Easy and Proven Way to Build Good Habits and Break Bad Ones*. Penguin Random House.

Csikszentmihalyi, M. (1990). *Flow: The Psychology of Optimal Experience*. Harper & Row.

Dweck, C. S. (2016). *Mindset: The New Psychology of Success*. Ballantine Books.

Kim, E. S., et al. (2022). "Sense of purpose in life and subsequent physical, behavioral, and psychosocial health: An outcome-wide approach. *The American Journal of Health Promotion, 36*(1), 137–147. pubmed.ncbi.nlm.nih.gov/34405718.

Lazar, S. W., et al. (2005). "Meditation experience is associated with increased cortical thickness." *NeuroReport, 16*(17), 1893–1897. pubmed.ncbi.nlm.nih.gov/16272874.

Mather, M. (2020). *The Science of Positivity: Stop Negative Thought Patterns by Changing Your Brain Chemistry*. Simon & Schuster.

Merzenich, M. M. (2013). *Soft-Wired: How the New Science of Brain Plasticity Can Change Your Life*. Parnassus Publishing.

Stanford Center on Longevity. (2022). "The new map of life." Stanford University. longevity.stanford.edu/the-new-map-of-life-report.

Chapter 6: The Biology of Authenticity: Your Cells Know When You're Lying to Yourself

Boehm, J. K., et al. (2011). "Heart health when life is satisfying: Evidence from the Whitehall II cohort study." *European Heart Journal, 32*(21), 2672–2679. doi.org/10.1093/eurheartj/ehr203.

Harvard T.H. Chan School of Public Health. (2011). "Satisfaction with daily life may protect against heart disease." hsph.harvard.edu/news/press-releases/job-satisfaction-heart-health.

Shirom, A., et al. (2008). "The Job Demand-Control-Support model and stress-related low-grade inflammatory responses among healthy employees: A longitudinal study." *Work & Stress, 22*(2), 138–152. doi.org/10.1080/02678370802180830.

Won, J., et al. (2021). "Evidence for exercise-related plasticity in functional and structural neural network connectivity." *Neuroscience & Biobehavioral Reviews*, 131, 923–940. doi.org/10.1016/j.neubiorev.2021.10.013.

Chapter 7: The Chemistry of Calm: From Hippie Wisdom to Harvard Research

Blackburn, E. H., & Epel, E. S. (2017). *The Telomere Effect: A Revolutionary Approach to Living Younger, Healthier, Longer*. Grand Central Publishing.

Davidson, R. J., & Lutz, A. (2008). "Buddha's brain: Neuroplasticity and meditation." *IEEE Signal Processing Magazine, 25*(1), 176–174. doi.org/10.1109/MSP.2008.4431873.

Davidson, R. J., et al. (2003). "Alterations in brain and immune function produced by mindfulness meditation." *Psychosomatic Medicine, 65*(4), 564–570. doi.org/10.1097/01.PSY.0000077505.67574.E3.

Kabat-Zinn, J. (2013). *Full Catastrophe Living: Using the Wisdom of Your Body and Mind to Face Stress, Pain, and Illness* (Revised Edition). Bantam Books.

Lazar, S. W., et al. (2005). "Meditation experience is associated with increased cortical thickness." *NeuroReport, 16*(17), 1893–1897. doi.org/10.1097/01.wnr.0000186598.66243.19.

Meditation Research Program. (2024). "The next wave of meditation research and training." Massachusetts General Hospital and Harvard Medical School. meditation.mgh.harvard.edu.

Chapter 8: Softening into Strength: The Science of Emotional Mastery

Atkins, P. W. B., & Stough, C. (2005). "Does emotional intelligence change with age?" Paper presented at the Society for Research in Adult Development Annual Conference, Atlanta, GA. researchgate.net/publication/234377636_Does_Emotional_Intelligence_change_with_age

Barraza, J. A., et al. (2022). "Oxytocin release increases with age and is associated with life satisfaction and prosocial behaviors." *Frontiers in Behavioral Neuroscience, 16*, 846234. doi.org/10.3389/fnbeh.2022.846234.

Carstensen, L. L., et al. (2011). "Emotional experience improves with age: Evidence based on over 10 years of experience sampling." *Psychology and Aging, 26*(1), 21–33. doi.org/10.1037/a0021285.

Chen, Y., & Peng, Y. (2016). "Emotional intelligence mediates the relationship between age and subjective well-being." *International Journal of Aging & Human Development, 83*(2), 91–107. doi.org/10.1177/0091415016648705.

Crockford, C., et al. (2018). "The role of oxytocin in social buffering: What do primate studies add?" *Current Topics in Behavioral Neurosciences, 35*, 155–173. doi.org/10.1007/7854_2017_12.

Dantzer, R., et al. (2018). "Resilience and immunity." *Brain, Behavior, and Immunity, 74*, 28–42. doi.org/10.1016/j.bbi.2018.08.010.

Dunietz, G. L., et al. (2024). "Oxytocin and women's health in midlife." *Journal of Endocrinology, 262*(1), e230396. doi.org/10.1530/JOE-23-0396.

Ebner, N. C., et al. (2015). "Oxytocin modulates meta-mood as a function of age and sex." *Frontiers in Aging Neuroscience, 7*, 175. doi.org/10.3389/fnagi.2015.00175.

Fabbri-Destro, M., & Rizzolatti, G. (2008). "Mirror neurons and mirror systems in monkeys and humans." *Physiology, 23*(3), 171–179. doi.org/10.1152/physiol.00004.2008.

Ferrari, P. F., & Coudé, G. (2018). "Mirror neurons, embodied emotions, and empathy." In K. Z. Meyza & E. Knapska (Eds.), *Neuronal Correlates of Empathy: From Rodent to Human*, (67–77). Elsevier Academic Press.

Goleman, D. (1998). "What makes a leader?: IQ and technical skills are important, but emotional intelligence is the sine qua non of leadership." *Harvard Business Review, 76*(6), 93–102. hbr.org/2004/01/what-makes-a-leader.

Murphy, M. L. M., Janicki-Deverts, D., & Cohen, S. (2018). "Receiving a hug is associated with the attenuation of negative mood that occurs on days with interpersonal conflict." *PLoS One, 13*(10), e0203522. doi.org/10.1371/journal.pone.0203522.

Samanez-Larkin, G. R., & Carstensen, L. L. (2011). "Socioemotional functioning and the aging brain." In J. Decety & J. T. Cacioppo (Eds.), *The Oxford Handbook of Social Neuroscience,* (507–521). Oxford University Press. doi.org/10.1093/oxfordhb/9780195342161.013.0034.

Wiltermuth, S. S., & Heath, C. (2009). "Synchrony and cooperation." *Psychological Science*, 20(1), 1–5. doi.org/10.1111/j.1467-9280.2008.02253.x.

Chapter 9: Wired to Connect: From Mirror Neurons to Belly Laughs

Alter, A. (2017). *Irresistible: The Rise of Addictive Technology and the Business of Keeping Us Hooked.* Penguin Press.

Bennett, M. P., & Lengacher, C. (2009). "Humor and laughter may influence health IV. Humor and immune function." *Evidence-Based Complementary and Alternative Medicine, 6*(2): 159–164. pmc.ncbi.nlm.nih.gov/articles/PMC2686627.

Bennett, M. P., et al. (2003). "The effect of mirthful laughter on stress and natural killer cell activity." *Alternative Therapies in Health and Medicine, 9*(2): 38–45. pubmed.ncbi.nlm.nih.gov/12652882.

Berk, L. S., et al. (2001). "Modulation of neuroimmune parameters during the eustress of humor-associated mirthful laughter." *Alternative Therapies in Health and Medicine, 7*(2): 62–72. pubmed.ncbi.nlm.nih.gov/11253418.

Berman, M. G., et al. (2008). "The cognitive benefits of interacting with nature." *Psychological Science, 19*(12): 1207–1212. pubmed.ncbi.nlm.nih.gov/19121124.

Davila Ross, M., Owren, M. J., & Zimmermann, E. (2009). "Reconstructing the evolution of laughter in great apes and humans." *Current Biology, 19*(13): 1106–1111. pubmed.ncbi.nlm.nih.gov/19500987.

Fredrickson, B. L., & Joiner, T. (2002). "Positive emotions trigger upward spirals toward emotional well-being." *Psychological Science,* *13*(2): 172–175. pubmed.ncbi.nlm.nih.gov/11934003.

Holt-Lunstad, J., et al. (2010). "Social relationships and mortality risk: A meta-analytic review." *PLoS Medicine,* *7*(7): e1000316. doi. org/10.1371/journal.pmed.1000316.

Holt-Lunstad, J., et al. (2015). "Loneliness and social isolation as risk factors for mortality: A meta-analytic review." *Perspectives on Psychological Science,* *10*(2): 227–237. pubmed.ncbi.nlm.nih. gov/25910392.

Horton, D., & Wohl, R. R. (1956). "Mass communication and para-social interaction: Observations on intimacy at a distance." *Psychiatry,* *19*(3): 215–229. pubmed.ncbi.nlm.nih.gov/13359569.

Janik, V. M., & Slater, P. J. B. (1998). "Context-specific use suggests that bottlenose dolphin signature whistles are cohesion calls." *Animal Behaviour,* *56*(4): 829–838. pubmed.ncbi.nlm.nih.gov/9790693.

Panksepp, J., & Burgdorf, J. (2003). "'Laughing' rats and the evolutionary antecedents of human joy?" *Physiology & Behavior,* *79*(3): 533–547. pubmed.ncbi.nlm.nih.gov/12954448.

Pantell, M., et al. (2013). "Social isolation: A predictor of mortality comparable to traditional clinical risk factors." *American Journal of Public Health,* *103*(11): 2056–2062. pmc.ncbi.nlm.nih.gov/articles/PMC3871270.

Rizzolatti, G., & Craighero, L. (2004). "The mirror-neuron system." *Annual Review of Neuroscience,* *27*, 169–192. pubmed.ncbi.nlm.nih. gov/15217330.

Sherman, L. E., et al. (2016). "The power of the like in adolescence: Effects of peer influence on neural and behavioral responses to social media." *Psychological Science,* *27*(7): 1027–1035. pubmed. ncbi.nlm.nih.gov/27247125.

Sinclair, D. A. (2019). *Lifespan: Why We Age—and Why We Don't Have To.* Atria Books.

Stephens, G. J., Silbert, L. J., & Hasson, U. (2010). "Speaker-listener neural coupling underlies successful communication." *Proceedings of the National Academy of Sciences USA,* *107*(32): 14425–14430. pubmed.ncbi.nlm.nih.gov/20660768.

Uncapher, M. R., & Wagner, A. D. (2018). "Minds and brains of media multitaskers: Current findings and future directions." *Proceedings of the National Academy of Sciences USA* 115(40): 9889–9896.

Winnick, M. (2016). "You touch your phone 2,617 times a day?!: Mobile touches: a dscout study on humans and their tech." *Medium.* medium.com/peoplenerds/putting-a-finger-on-our-phone-obsession-d65734181dc7.

Yang, Y. C., et al. (2016). "Social relationships and physiological determinants of longevity across the human life span." *Proceedings of the National Academy of Sciences USA*, 113(3): 578–583. pubmed.ncbi.nlm.nih.gov/26729882.

Chapter 10: The Currency of Compound Experience: Investing in Your Second Prime

AARP & Economist Intelligence Unit. (2019). "The Longevity Economy Outlook: How People Age 50 and Older Are Fueling Economic Growth, Stimulating Jobs, and Creating Opportunities for All." AARP. www.reserveinc.org/files/PDFs/Longevity%20Economy%20Outlook%20-%20AARP%20-%2003_2020.pdf

Abouzahr, K., et al. (2018, June 6). "Why women-owned startups are a better bet." Boston Consulting Group & MassChallenge. www.bcg.com/publications/2018/why-women-owned-startups-are-better-bet.

Azoulay, P., et al. (2020). "Age and high-growth entrepreneurship." *American Economic Review: Insights*, 2(1), 65–82. doi.org/10.1257/aeri.20180582.

Bersin, J. & Chamorro-Premuzic, T. (2019). "The case for hiring older workers." *Harvard Business Review.* hbr.org/2019/09/the-case-for-hiring-older-workers.

Credit Suisse Research Institute (2023). *Global Wealth Report 2023.* www.ubs.com/global/en/family-office-uhnw/reports/global-wealth-report-2023/_jcr_content/mainpar/toplevelgrid_5684475_1708633751/col1/innergrid/xcol1/actionbutton_copy_co.1784379955.file/PS9jb250ZW50L-2RhbS9hc3NldHMvd20vZ2xvYmFsL2l0Zy9nbG9iYWwtYWwtZm-

FtaWx5LW9mZmljZS9kb2NzL2d3ci0yMDIzLWVuLTIuc-
GRm/gwr-2023-en-2.pdf

Deloitte Center for Health Solutions. (2019). "The future of aging:
What impact might the expansion of health span have on society?" Deloitte Insights. www.deloitte.com/us/en/insights/indus-
try/health-care/future-of-aging-aging-population-and-health-
care-industry.html

Department of Economic and Social Affairs: Population Division.
(2022). "World population prospects 2024." United Nations.
population.un.org/wpp.

Economist Intelligence Unit (2023). "The longevity economy: Opportunities in the silver market." graphics.eiu.com/upload/eb/
Axa_Longevity-EIU_Web.pdf.

Fairlie, R., Desai, S., & Herrmann, A. J. (2019). "2018 National Report
on Early-Stage Entrepreneurship in the United States." Kauffman Indicators of Entrepreneurship. indicators.kauffman.
org/wp-content/uploads/sites/2/2019/09/National_Report_
Sept_2019.pdf

Hiscox. (2019). *2019 Hiscox Ageism in the Workplace Study*. Hiscox USA.
www.hiscox.com/documents/2019-Hiscox-Ageism-Work-
place-Study.pdf.

Munnell, A. H. (2025, April 15). "Will the average retirement age keep
rising?" Center for Retirement Research at Boston College. crr.
bc.edu/will-the-average-retirement-age-keep-rising/

National Center for Health Statistics (2023). "Life expectancy." Centers for Disease Control and Prevention. cdc.gov/nchs/fastats/
life-expectancy.htm.

OECD. (2019). "Working better with age: Ageing and employment
policies." OECD Publishing. doi.org/10.1787/c4d4f66a-en

PricewaterhouseCoopers. (2018). "Golden Age Index 2018: Unlocking
a potential $3.5 trillion prize from longer working lives." PwC.
www.pwc.com/gx/en/news-room/docs/pwc-golden-age-index.
pdf

PricewaterhouseCoopers. (2018). *Golden Age Index: Unlocking the Economic
Potential of Older Workers*. pwc.co.uk/economic-services/gold-
en-age/golden-age-index-2018-final-sanitised.pdf.

Stanford Center on Longevity. (2022). "The new map of life." Stanford University. longevity.stanford.edu/the-new-map-of-life-report.

U.S. Bureau of Labor Statistics. (2024). "Labor force statistics from the current population survey." U.S. Department of Labor. bls.gov/cps.

Chapter 11: From Target Market to Market Maker: Flipping the Script on Aging Narratives

AARP. (2019). "Media image landscape: Age representation in online images." AARP Research. www.aarp.org/pri/topics/aging-experience/age-representation-in-online-media-images/

Ace Metrix. (2016, August 24). "Ad of the Week: The Iron Nun inspires us all in Nike's 'Unlimited Youth.'" Ace Metrix Insights. www.acemetrix.com/insights/blog/ad-of-the-week-the-iron-nun-inspires-us-all-in-nikes-unlimited-youth/

Campaign Media Awards. (2025). "L'Oréal: YOU Look Great." Campaign Media Awards, Haymarket Media Group. www.campaignmediaawards.com/finalists/loreal-you-look-great-8qql2ez36q73l4y.

Celebre, A., & Waggoner Denton, A. (2014). "The good, the bad, and the ugly of the Dove Campaign for Real Beauty." *In-Mind Magazine*, 2(19). www.in-mind.org/article/the-good-the-bad-and-the-ugly-of-the-dove-campaign-for-real-beauty

Fairlie, R. & Desai, S. (2021). "National report on early-stage entrepreneurship in the United States: 2020." Ewing Marion Kauffman Foundation. www.kauffman.org/reports/early-stage-entrepreneurship-national-trends-2020.

Godin, S. (2023). *This Is Marketing: You Can't Be Seen Until You Learn to See.* Portfolio.

Griesel, D. (2024). *Silver Disobedience: A Philosophy on Aging and Living Agelessly.* Silver Disobedience Inc.

Ipsos. (2024). "Advertising for Better Representation." Ipsos VIEWS. www.ipsos.com/sites/default/files/ct/publication/documents/2024-07/Advertising_for_Better_Representation.pdf.

Kakulla, B. (2024). "The Longevity economy outlook." AARP Research. aarp.org/research/topics/economics/info-2019/longevi-ty-economy-outlook.html.

Louis-Dreyfus, J. (Host). (2021–present). *Wiser Than Me with Julia Lou-is-Dreyfus* (Audio podcast.) Lemonada Media. lemonadamedia. com/show/wiser-than-me.

MARC Group. (2021, February 22). "Global anti-aging market report and forecast 2021–2026." ResearchAndMarkets. www.business-wire.com/news/home/20210222005466/en/Global-Anti-Ag-ing-Market-2021-to-2026---Featuring-Allergan-Beiersdorf-Unile-ver-Among-Others---ResearchAndMarkets.com.

McKinsey & Company. (2020, April 28). "Personalizing the customer experience: Driving differentiation in retail." McKinsey & Com-pany. www.mckinsey.com/industries/retail/our-insights/person-alizing-the-customer-experience-driving-differentiation-in-retail.

Ng, R., Indran, N., & Liu, L. (2024). "Advocating for older adults in the age of social media: Strategies to achieve peak engagement on Twitter." *JMIR Aging*, 7, e49608. doi.org/10.2196/49608.

Nyad, D. (2015). *Find a Way: The Inspiring Story of One Woman's Pursuit of a Lifelong Dream*. Knopf.

Schøtt, T., et al. (2017). "GEM special topic report: Senior entre-preneurship 2016/2017." Global Entrepreneurship Research Association. gemconsortium.org/report/gem-2016-2017-re-port-on-senior-entrepreneurship.

Unstereotype Alliance. (2024). "Inclusion = Income: The business case for inclusive advertising. UN Women & Saïd Business School." www.unstereotypealliance.org/sites/default/files/2024-09/INCLUSIVE%20ADVERTISING%20%28Business%20case%29%20WEB.pdf.

US Masters Swimming. (2024). "Registration statistics 1987–current." Guide to Operations. www.usms.org/-/media/usms/pdfs/guide%20to%20operations%20-%20gto/lmsc%20manage-ment/reg_historical_stats.pdf.

Wikipedia. (2025). "Source credibility." In *Wikipedia*. Retrieved June 11, 2025, from en.wikipedia.org/wiki/Source_credibility

Chapter 12: Beyond X and Y: Reimagining Biological Differences in Our Second Prime

Allard, E. S., & Kensinger, E. A. (2014). "Age-related differences in neural recruitment during the use of cognitive reappraisal and selective attention as emotion regulation strategies." *Frontiers in Psychology, 5,* 296. doi.org/10.3389/fpsyg.2014.00296.

Aviv, A., et al. (2005). "The longevity gender gap: Are telomeres the explanation?" *Science of Aging Knowledge Environment, 2005*(23), pe16. doi.org/10.1126/sageke.2005.23.pe16.

Barrett, E. L., & Richardson, D. S. (2011). "Sex differences in telomeres and lifespan." *Aging Cell, 10*(6), 913–921. doi.org/10.1111/j.1474-9726.2011.00741.x.

Carstensen, L. L. (2006). "The influence of a sense of time on human development." *Science, 312*(5782), 1913–1915. doi.org/10.1126/science.1127488.

Cassidy, B. S., et al. (2013). "Valence-based age differences in medial prefrontal activity during impression formation." *Social Cognitive and Affective Neuroscience, 8*(7), 853–860. pubmed.ncbi.nlm.nih.gov/23998453.

Diaz Granados, C. A., et al. (2014). "Efficacy of high-dose versus standard-dose influenza vaccine in older adults." *New England Journal of Medicine, 371*(7), 635–645. doi.org/10.1056/NEJMoa1315727.

Fusar-Poli, P., et al. (2009). "Functional atlas of emotional faces processing: A voxel-based meta-analysis." *Journal of Psychiatry & Neuroscience, 34*(6), 418–432. jpn.ca/content/34/6/418.

Gardner, M., et al. (2014). "Gender and telomere length: Systematic review and meta-analysis." *Experimental Gerontology, 51,* 15–27. doi.org/10.1016/j.exger.2013.12.004.

Giefing-Kröll, C., et al. (2015). "How sex and age affect immune responses, susceptibility to infections, and response to vaccination." *Aging Cell, 14*(3), 309–321. doi.org/10.1111/acel.12326.

Gunning-Dixon, F. M., et al. (2009). "Aging of cerebral white matter: A review of MRI findings." *International Journal of Geriatric Psychiatry, 24*(2), 109–117. doi.org/10.1002/gps.2087.

Holt-Lunstad, J., Smith, T. B., & Layton, J. B. (2010). "Social relationships and mortality risk: A meta-analytic review." *PLOS Medicine,* 7(7), e1000316. doi.org/10.1371/journal.pmed.1000316.

Klein, S. L., & Flanagan, K. L. (2016). "Sex differences in immune responses." *Nature Reviews Immunology, 16*(10), 626–638. doi. org/10.1038/nri.2016.90.

Kryla-Lighthall, N., & Mather, M. (2009). "The role of cognitive control in older adults' emotional well-being." In V. L. Bengtson et al. (Eds.), *Handbook of Theories of Aging,* second ed. (323–344). Springer.

Kuiper, J. S., et al. (2015). "Social relationships and risk of dementia: A systematic review and meta-analysis of longitudinal cohort studies." *Ageing Research Reviews, 22,* 39–57. doi.org/10.1016/j. arr.2015.04.006.

Mather, M., & Carstensen, L. L. (2005). "Aging and motivated cognition: The positivity effect in attention and memory." *Trends in Cognitive Sciences, 9*(10), 496–502. doi.org/10.1016/j. tics.2005.08.005.

McArdle, J. J., Ferrer-Caja, E., Hamagami, F., & Woodcock, R. W. (2002). "Comparative longitudinal structural analyses of the growth and decline of multiple intellectual abilities over the life span." *Developmental Psychology, 38*(1), 115–142. doi. org/10.1037/0012-1649.38.1.115.

Pennebaker, J. W., & Chung, C. K. (2011). "Expressive writing and its links to mental and physical health." In H. S. Friedman (Ed.), *Oxford Handbook of Health Psychology* (417–437). Oxford University Press. doi.org/10.1093/oxfordhb/9780195342819.013.0018.

Ruffman, T., Henry, J. D., Livingstone, V., & Phillips, L. H. (2008). "A meta-analytic review of emotion recognition and aging: Implications for neuropsychological models of aging." *Neuroscience & Biobehavioral Reviews, 32*(4), 863–881. doi.org/10.1016/j.neubiorev.2008.01.001.

Vaillant, G. E. (2012). *Triumphs of Experience: The Men of the Harvard Grant Study.* Harvard University Press.

Vardeny, O., et al. (2018). "Decreased immune responses to influenza vaccination in patients with heart failure." *Journal of Cardiac Failure, 24*(11), 762–766. pmc.ncbi.nlm.nih.gov/articles/PMC2696231.

Waldinger, R. J., & Schulz, M. S. (2023). *The Good Life: Lessons from the World's Longest Scientific Study of Happiness.* Simon & Schuster.

Zalli, A., et al. (2014). "Shorter telomeres with high telomerase activity are associated with raised allostatic load and impoverished psychosocial resources." *Proceedings of the National Academy of Sciences, 111*(12), 4519–4524. doi.org/10.1073/pnas.1322145111.

Chapter 13: Pretty Rebellious: The Revolution Against Age-Based Beauty

Bakkila, B. (2016). "Ashley Graham makes history as the first size-16 model to cover *Sports Illustrated*: 'This is going to change my life forever.'" *People.* people.com/style/ashley-graham-makes-history-as-the-first-size-16-model-to-cover-sports-illustrated-this-is-going-to-change-my-life-forever.

Blackham, A. (2020, March 7). "Women, age discrimination and work." *Pursuit* (University of Melbourne). pursuit.unimelb.edu.au/articles/women-age-discrimination-and-work.

Dove & Edelman Intelligence. (2016). "The Dove Global Beauty and Confidence Report." Unilever. www.unilever.com/files/6d9ddfad-f03b-46cd-92a8-837c85023a15/dove-infographic-pdf.

Dove. (2016). "Our research." Unilever. dove.com/us/en/stories/about-dove/our-research.html.

Etcoff, N., et al. (2004). "The real truth about beauty: A global report: Findings of the global study on women, beauty and well-being." Dove, a Unilever Beauty Brand. clubofamsterdam.com/contentarticles/52%20Beauty/dove_white_paper_final.pdf.

Grimm, J., & Grimm, W. (1812/1884). *Household Tales* (M. Hunt, Trans.; 1st English ed.). George Bell & Sons. Project Gutenberg. www.gutenberg.org/files/5314/5314-h/5314-h.htm.

Herbison, M. (2015, September 15). "Target embraces diversity with new size 16 mannequins." *Marketing Magazine*. www.marketing-mag.com.au/news/target-embraces-diversity-new-size-16-man-nequins/.

Hilmantel, R. (2016, February 14). :Sports Illustrated Swimsuit Issue cover star Ashley Graham: Stop labeling women 'plus-size.'" *TIME*. time.com/4224444/sports-illustrated-swimsuit-issue-cov-er-model-ashley-graham-interview/

Hofmeier, S. M., et al. (2016). "Body image, aging, and identity in women over 50: The Gender and Body Image (GABI) Study." *Journal of Women & Aging, 29*(1), 3–14. doi.org/10.1080/0895284 1.2015.1065140.

Kakulla, B. (2024). "The Longevity economy outlook." AARP Research. aarp.org/research/topics/economics/info-2019/longevi-ty-economy-outlook.html.

Ko, H. J., et al. (2019). "Transitions to older adulthood: Exploring midlife women's narratives regarding purpose in life." *Journal of Positive Psychology and Wellbeing, 3*(2), 137–152. journalppw.com/index.php/jppw/article/view/36/34.

Ovid. (2004). *Metamorphoses: A New Translation*. C. Martin, Trans. W.W. Norton & Company.

Syropoulos, H. J. (2023). "Coming to terms with invisibility and age-ism." IBX Insights. insights.ibx.com/coming-to-terms-with-invis-ibility-and-ageism.

Westwood, S. (2023). "'It's the not being seen that is most tiresome': Older women, invisibility and social (in)justice." *Women's Studies International Forum, 98*, 102729. pubmed.ncbi.nlm.nih.gov/37097812.

Chapter 14: The Power of Three: Autonomy, Agency, and the Art of Optimistic Living

Amaral, A. S., et al. (2022). "Healthcare decision-making capacity in old age: A qualitative study." *Frontiers in Psychology, 13*, 1024967. doi.org/10.3389/fpsyg.2022.1024967

Cerino, E. S., et al. (2024). "Perceived control across the adult lifespan: Longitudinal changes in global control and daily stressor control." *Developmental Psychology,* 60(1), 45–58. pubmed.ncbi.nlm.nih.gov/37917487.

Cornwell, E. Y., & Waite, L. J. (2009). "Social disconnectedness, perceived isolation, and health among older adults." *Journal of Health and Social Behavior,* 50(1), 31–48. pubmed.ncbi.nlm.nih.gov/19413133.

Diehl, M., Coyle, N., & Labouvie-Vief, G. (1998). "Age and sex differences in strategies of coping and defense across the life span. *Psychology and Aging,* 11(1), 127–139. pubmed.ncbi.nlm.nih.gov/8726378.

Heintzelman, S. J., & Luger, T. (2021). "Experiences of solitude in adulthood and old age: The role of autonomy." *International Journal of Behavioral Development,* 45(5), 413–423. doi.org/10.1177/01650254221117498

Infurna, F. J., et al. (2011). "Long-term antecedents and outcomes of perceived control." *Psychology and Aging,* 26(4), 924–934. pubmed.ncbi.nlm.nih.gov/21517184.

James, P., et al. (2019). "Optimism and Healthy Aging in Women." *American Journal of Preventative Medicine.* 56(1):116–124. doi:10.1016/j.amepre.2018.07.037.

Jenkins, A., & Mostafa, T. (2015). "The effects of learning on wellbeing for older adults in England." *Ageing and Society,* 35(10), 2053–2070. cambridge.org/core/journals/ageing-and-society/article/effects-of-learning-on-wellbeing-for-older-adults-in-england/55134CB9C0B61D48BD6D10786CA26502.

Jusung Lee, K., White, K., & Dalton, V. K. (2025). "Mental distress among females following 2021 abortion restrictions in Texas." *JAMA Network Open,* 8(5), e259576. doi.org/10.1001/jamanetworkopen.2025.9576

Leanos, S., et al. (2020). "The impact of learning multiple real-world skills on cognitive abilities and functional independence in healthy older adults." *The Journals of Gerontology: Series B,* 75(6), 1155–1169. pubmed.ncbi.nlm.nih.gov/31201426.

Lee, C. C., et al. (2023). "The impact of living arrangements and social capital on the wellbeing of the elderly." *Healthcare*, 11(14), Article 2050. doi.org/10.3390/healthcare11142050

Lee, L. O., et al. (2019). "Optimism is associated with exceptional longevity in 2 epidemiologic cohorts of men and women." *Proceedings of the National Academy of Sciences, 116*(37), 18357–18362. pubmed.ncbi.nlm.nih.gov/31451635.

Masters, K. S., & Hooker, S. A. (2013). "Religiousness/spirituality, cardiovascular disease, and cancer: Cultural integration for health research and intervention." *Journal of Consulting and Clinical Psychology, 81*(2), 206–216. pubmed.ncbi.nlm.nih.gov/23148874.

Moilanen, T., & Kangasniemi, M. (2021). "Older people's perceived autonomy in residential care: An integrative review." *Nursing Ethics*, 28(3), 414–434. doi.org/10.1177/0969733020948115

Nakamura, J. S., et al. (2022). "Reduced epigenetic age in older adults who volunteer." *Psychoneuroendocrinology, 148*, 106000. doi. org/10.1016/j.psyneuen.2022.106000

Narushima, M., Liu, J., & Diestelkamp, N. (2018). "Lifelong learning in active ageing discourse: Its conserving effect on wellbeing, health and vulnerability." *Ageing and Society, 38*(4), 651–675. pubmed. ncbi.nlm.nih.gov/29551843.

Opsasnick, L. A., et al. (2024). "Epigenome-wide mediation analysis of the relationship between psychosocial stress and cardiometabolic risk factors in the Health and Retirement Study (HRS)." *Clinical Epigenetics*, 16, Article 180. clinicalepigeneticsjournal.biomedcentral.com/articles/10.1186/s13148-024-01799-4

Pargament, K. I., et al. (2001). "The many methods of religious coping: Development and initial validation of the RCOPE." *Journal of Clinical Psychology, 57*(4), 519–543. pubmed.ncbi.nlm.nih. gov/10775045/

Pirutinsky, S., et al. (2011). "Does negative religious coping accompany, precede, or follow depression among Orthodox Jews?" *Journal of Affective Disorders, 132*(3), 401–405. pubmed.ncbi.nlm.nih. gov/21439650.

Rentscher, K. E., et al. (2019). "Chronic stress exposure and daily stress appraisals relate to biological aging marker p16^INK4a." *Psychoneuroendocrinology*, 102, 139–148. doi.org/10.1016/j.psyn-euen.2018.12.006

Richardson, T., Elliott, P., & Roberts, R. (2017). "A longitudinal study of financial difficulties and mental health in a national sample of British undergraduate students." *Community Mental Health Journal*, 53(3), 344–354. pubmed.ncbi.nlm.nih.gov/27473685.

Russo, M., et al. (2018). "Boundary management permeability and relationship satisfaction in dualearner couples: The asymmetrical gender effect." *Frontiers in Psychology*, 9, Article 1723. doi.org/10.3389/fpsyg.2018.01723

Toyama, M., & Fuller, H. R. (2021). "Longitudinal associations between perceived control and health for American and Japanese aging adults." *The Gerontologist*, 61(6), 917–929. doi.org/10.1093/geront/gnaa135

Turunen, E., & Hiilamo, H. (2014). "Health effects of indebtedness: A systematic review." *BMC Public Health*, 14, 489. pubmed.ncbi.nlm.nih.gov/24885280.

Windsor, T. D., Curtis, R. G., & Luszcz, M. A. (2015). "Perceived control moderates the effects of functional limitation on older adults' social activity: Findings from the Australian Longitudinal Study of Ageing." *Journal of Gerontology: Series B*, 70(4), 592–603. pubmed.ncbi.nlm.nih.gov/26424833.

Windsor, T. D., WiltonHarding, B., & Sabatini, S. (2024). "Daily dynamics of awareness of aging and basic psychological need satisfaction and frustration in middle and older adulthood." *The Journals of Gerontology: Series B*, 79(4), gbae010. doi.org/10.1093/geronb/gbae010

Yeo, J., & Lee, Y. G. (2019). "Understanding the association between perceived financial well-being and life satisfaction among older adults: Does social capital play a role?" *Journal of Family and Economic Issues*, 40(4), 592–608. doi.org/10.1007/s10834-019-09634-2

Chapter 15: Your Inner Pharmacy: Harnessing Microbiome Magic

Arboleya, S., et al. (2016). "Gut bifidobacteria populations in human health and aging." *Frontiers in Microbiology, 7*, 1204. doi. org/10.3389/fmicb.2016.01204.

Azuma, T., et al. (2004). "Gastric leptin and *Helicobacter pylori* infection." *Gut,* 53(7), 918–922. pmc.ncbi.nlm.nih.gov/articles/ PMC1728440.

Baik, H. W., & Russell, R. M. (1999). "Vitamin B12 deficiency in the elderly." *Annual Review of Nutrition, 19*, 357–377. doi.org/10.1146/ annurev.nutr.19.1.357.

Björklund, M., et al. (2012). "Gut microbiota of healthy elderly NSAID users is selectively modified with the administration of *Lactobacillus acidophilus* NCFM and lactitol." *Age, 34*, 987–999. doi. org/10.1007/s11357-011-9294-5.

David, L. A., et al. (2014). "Diet rapidly and reproducibly alters the human gut microbiome." *Nature, 505*(7484), 559–563. doi. org/10.1038/nature12820.

Dinan, T. G., & Cryan, J. F. (2017). "Brain-gut-microbiota axis—Mood, metabolism and behaviour." *Nature Reviews Gastroenterology & Hepatology, 14*(2), 69–70. doi.org/10.1038/nrgastro.2016.200.

Erny, D., Hrabě de Angelis, A. L., & Prinz, M. (2017). "Communicating systems in the body: How microbiota and microglia cooperate." *Immunology, 150*(1), 7–15. doi.org/10.1111/imm.12645.

Gershon, M. D. (2013). "5-Hydroxytryptamine (serotonin) in the gastrointestinal tract." *Current Opinion in Endocrinology, Diabetes, and Obesity, 20*(1), 14–21. doi.org/10.1097/MED.0b013e32835bc703.

Gomez-Pinilla, P. J., et al. (2011). "Changes in interstitial cells of cajal with age in the human stomach and colon." *Neurogastroenterology & Motility, 23*(1), 36–44. doi.org/10.1111/j.1365-2982.2010.01590.x.

Gutierrez, D., et al. (2021). "Circadian rhythms and the gut microbiome synchronize the host's metabolic response to diet." *Cell Metabolism,* 34(7), 1012-1027. doi.org/10.1016/j.cmet.2021.03.015

Jackson, M. A., et al. (2016). "Signatures of early frailty in the gut microbiota." *Genome Medicine, 8*(1), 8. doi.org/10.1186/s13073-016-0262-7.

Johnson, K.V.A., & Foster, K.R. (2021). "Gut microbiome composition and diversity are related to human personality traits." *Human Microbiobe Journal.* 2020 Mar; 98, 361–371. pubmed.ncbi.nlm.nih.gov/34435164/.

Kim, H. N., et al. (2020). "Emotional well-being and gut microbiome profiles by enterotype." *Scientific Reports*, 10, Article 20736. doi.org/10.1038/s41598-020-77673-z

Kim, S., & Jazwinski, S. M. (2018). "The gut microbiota and healthy aging: A mini-review." *Gerontology, 64*(6), 513–520. doi.org/10.1159/000490615.

La-Ongkham, O., et al. (2020). "Age-related changes in the gut microbiota and the core gut microbiome of healthy Thai humans." *3 Biotech, 10*, 276. pubmed.ncbi.nlm.nih.gov/32537376.

Laugier, R., et al. (1991). "Changes in pancreatic exocrine secretion with age: Pancreatic exocrine secretion does decrease in the elderly." *Digestion*, 50(3–4), 202–11. doi.org/10.1159/000200762

Li, Q., et al. (2007). "Forest bathing enhances human natural killer activity and expression of anti-cancer proteins." *International Journal of Immunopathology and Pharmacology*, 20(2 Suppl 2), 3–8. doi.org/10.1177/03946320070200S202

Liu, P., et al. (2021). "Gut microbiota: Critical controller and intervention target in brain aging and cognitive impairment" *Frontiers in Aging Neuroscience*, 13, 671142. doi.org/10.3389/fnagi.2021.671142

Madison, A., et al. (2019). "Stress, depression, diet, and the gut microbiota: Human–bacteria interactions at the core of psychoneuroimmunology and nutrition." *Current Opinion in Behavioral Sciences*, 28, 105–110. doi.org/10.1016/j.cobeha.2019.01.011

Maseda, D., & Ricciotti, E. (2020). "NSAID: Gut Microbiota Interactions." *Frontiers in Pharmacology*, 11, 1153. doi.org/10.3389/fphar.2020.01153

Mayer, E. A., Tillisch, K., & Gupta, A. (2015). "Gut/brain axis and the microbiota." *Journal of Clinical Investigation, 125*(3), 926–938. doi. org/10.1172/JCI76304.

McDonald, D., et al. (2018). "American gut: An open platform for citizen science microbiome research." *American Society for Microbiology Journals, 3*(3), e00031–18. journals.asm.org/doi/10.1128/msystems.00031-18.

O'Mahony, S. M., et al. (2015). "Serotonin, tryptophan metabolism and the brain-gut-microbiome axis." *Behavioural Brain Research, 277*, 32–48. doi.org/10.1016/j.bbr.2014.07.027.

O'Toole, P. W., & Jeffery, I. B. (2015). "Gut microbiota and aging." *Science, 350*(6265), 1214–1215. doi.org/10.1126/science.aac8469.

Perez-Pardo, P., et al. (2017). "The gut-brain axis in Parkinson's disease: Possibilities for food-based therapies." *European Journal of Pharmacology, 817*, 86–95. pubmed.ncbi.nlm.nih.gov/28549787.

Rogers, M. A., et al. (2016). "The influence of non-steroidal anti-inflammatory drugs on the gut microbiome." *Clinical Microbiology and Infection*, 22(2), 178.e1-178.e9. doi.org/10.1016/j. cmi.2015.10.003

Salazar, N., et al. (2014). "The human intestinal microbiome at extreme ages of life: Dietary intervention as a way to counteract alterations." *Frontiers in Genetics, 5*, 406. doi.org/10.3389/fgene.2014.00406.

Schnorr, S. L., et al. (2014). "Gut microbiome of the Hadza hunter-gatherers." *Nature Communications, 5*, 3654. doi.org/10.1038/ncomms4654.

Valdes, A. M., et al. (2018). "Role of the gut microbiota in nutrition and health." *British Medical Journal, 361*, k2179. doi.org/10.1136/bmj.k2179.

Yano, J. M., et al. (2015). "Indigenous bacteria from the gut microbiota regulate host serotonin biosynthesis." *Cell, 161*(2), 264–276. doi. org/10.1016/j.cell.2015.02.047.

Chapter 16: Glimmers and Wonder: The Gift of Enhanced Joy!

Barrett, L. F., & Bliss-Moreau, E. (2009). "Affect as a psychological primitive." *Advances in Experimental Social Psychology, 41*, 167–218. doi.org/10.1016/S0065-2601(08)00404-8.

Carstensen, L. L. (2006). "The influence of a sense of time on human development." *Science, 312*(5782), 1913–1915. doi.org/10.1126/science.1127488.

Carstensen, L. L. et al. (2011). "Emotional experience improves with age: Evidence based on over 10 years of experience sampling." *Psychology and Aging, 26*(1), 21–33. doi.org/10.1037/a0021285.

Charles, S. T., & Carstensen, L. L. (2010). "Social and emotional aging." *Annual Review of Psychology, 61*, 383–409. doi.org/10.1146/annurev.psych.093008.100448.

Dana, D. (2018). *The Polyvagal Theory in Therapy: Engaging the Rhythm of Regulation.* W.W. Norton & Company.

Dana, D. (2021). *Anchored: How to Befriend Your Nervous System Using Polyvagal Theory.* Sounds True.

English, T., & Carstensen, L. L. (2014). "Selective narrowing of social networks across adulthood is associated with improved emotional experience in daily life." *International Journal of Behavioral Development, 38*(2), 195–202. doi.org/10.1177/0165025413515404.

Fredrickson, B. L. (2013). "Positive emotions broaden and build." *Advances in Experimental Social Psychology, 47*, 1–53. doi.org/10.1016/B978-0-12-407236-7.00001-2.

Fredrickson, B. L., & Joiner, T. (2018). "Reflections on positive emotions and upward spirals." *Perspectives on Psychological Science, 13*(2), 194–199. pubmed.ncbi.nlm.nih.gov/29592643.

Garland, E. L. et al. (2010). "Upward spirals of positive emotions counter downward spirals of negativity: Insights from the broaden-and-build theory and affective neuroscience on the treatment of emotion dysfunctions and deficits in psychopathology." *Clinical Psychology Review, 30*(7), 849-864. doi.org/10.1016/j.cpr.2010.03.002.

Hölzel, B. K. et al. (2011). "Mindfulness practice leads to increases in regional brain gray matter density." *Psychiatry Research: Neuroimaging, 191*(1), 36–43. doi.org/10.1016/j.pscychresns.2010.08.006.

Isaacowitz, D. M. et al. (2006). "Selective preference in visual fixation away from negative images in old age?: An eye-tracking study." *Psychology and Aging, 21*(1), 40–48. doi.org/10.1037/0882-7974.21.1.40.

Mather, M. et al. (2016). "Norepinephrine ignites local hotspots of neuronal excitation: How arousal amplifies selectivity in perception and memory." B*ehavioral and Brain Sciences, 39*, e200. doi.org/10.1017/S0140525X15000667.

Mather, M., & Carstensen, L. L. (2005). "Aging and motivated cognition: The positivity effect in attention and memory." *Trends in Cognitive Sciences, 9*(10), 496–502. doi.org/10.1016/j.tics.2005.08.005.

Reed, A. E., Chan, L., & Mikels, J. A. (2014). "Meta-analysis of the age-related positivity effect: Age differences in preferences for positive over negative information." *Psychology and Aging, 29*(1), 1–15. doi.org/10.1037/a0035194.

Scheibe, S., & Carstensen, L. L. (2010). "Emotional aging: Recent findings and future trends." *The Journals of Gerontology: Series B, 65B*(2), 135–144. doi.org/10.1093/geronb/gbp132.

Stellar, J. E. et al. (2015). "Positive affect and markers of inflammation: Discrete positive emotions predict lower levels of inflammatory cytokines." *Emotion, 15*(2), 129–133. doi.org/10.1037/emo0000033.

Urry, H. L., & Gross, J. J. (2010). "Emotion regulation in older age." *Current Directions in Psychological Science, 19*(6), 352–357. doi.org/10.1177/0963721410388395.

Waldinger, R. J., & Schulz, M. S. (2010). "What's love got to do with it?: Social functioning, perceived health, and daily happiness in married octogenarians." *Psychology and Aging, 25*(2), 422–431. doi.org/10.1037/a0019087.

Waldinger, R. J., & Schulz, M. S. (2016). "The long reach of nurturing family environments: Links with midlife emotion-regulatory styles and late-life security in intimate relationships." *Psychological Science,* *27*(11), 1443–1450. doi.org/10.1177/0956797616661556.

Zaki, J., & Williams, W. C. (2013). "Interpersonal emotion regulation." *Emotion,* *13*(5), 803–810. doi.org/10.1037/a0033839.

Acknowledgments

Every book is a journey, and this one began with two extraordinary human beings who make my life infinitely richer. To my husband, Lance—thank you for believing in me even when I disappeared into late-night writing sessions, holding space when I needed it, and never once questioning whether this inconvenient dream was worth pursuing. And to my beautiful son, Hudson, you are my heart walking outside my body. May you grow to love every stage of your life, embracing each chapter with the same curiosity and joy you show me daily.

To my mom, who has redefined what it means to flourish in a Third Prime—you've shown me that our capacity for growth never diminishes, only grows stronger. Your evolution continues to inspire me.

To the extraordinary and thoughtful people who are my work family in healthcare—the culture of love and support with my intelligent colleagues, brilliant researchers, physicians, and professionals who have taught me on every level—your dedication and commitment to science and caring deeply for others have shaped my career and my understanding of what it means to live with purpose. Your wisdom flows through these pages in countless ways.

To my community of supporters—some who walked alongside me daily and others whose profound influence shaped the very foundation of who I am. To the mentors, teachers, and luminaries who bring light and inspiration, who may never know how deeply their wisdom altered my path, your impact on me echoes throughout these pages. To my dear friends—the Jennas, Mimi, Dennis, Greg, Bruce, Angie, Elizabeth, Abby, Debbie, Kristie, Tracey, Lily, and Bri—your love, wisdom, and support have shown me what impact truly looks like. To Kristi, Dawn, Anissia, the Jenns, Jamie,

Yolanda, Penny, Amy, and Sadra, who listened patiently when I said I wanted to have a podcast and write a book; you encouraged me, read drafts, and offered inspiration precisely when needed. And also to Jade, Pam, Heather, Joy, and Christine, who appeared as angels to champion this work.

Some influences transcend daily interaction—to those whose books, speeches, or brief but powerful moments of connection fundamentally altered how I see the world and myself, thank you for proving that transformation doesn't always require proximity, only openness to receive the gift of another's truth.

For each roadblock and challenge that shaped me, thank you for teaching me that the obstacle is indeed the way.

To Sue, my first editor, who gave me hope, thank you for fearlessly holding the slop bucket of my earliest drafts and seeing potential where I saw only chaos. And to Marley, who masterfully untangled my thoughts, your insight transformed this manuscript.

Finally, to everyone from every generation who has ever questioned the narrative around aging, this is for you. To the young person afraid of what lies ahead, those amid transition, and those already embracing their Second, Third, or Fourth Prime—may we collectively rewrite what it means to grow older in this world, not as a descent into irrelevance, but as an ascent into our most authentic, powerful, and beautiful selves with each passing year.

With profound gratitude,

Gretchen

About the Author

Gretchen Terry-Leonard has spent over three decades asking the kinds of questions that reframe assumptions and unlock possibilities in her biotech professional and wellness specialist career—and that's precisely what makes her so effective. Working at the intersection of health, science, AI, and health equity, her professional career has been shaped by a deep commitment to making healthcare more humane, equitable, and forward-looking.

In her current role, she created and leads I'M IN, a nationwide initiative focused on creating structural change in healthcare systems. Under her leadership, I'M IN has established Health Equity Fellowships at top-tier institutions across the United States. Through this work, Gretchen builds meaningful alliances across neurology, oncology, and fertility—spaces where innovation and impact must go hand in hand. She's known for convening people tired of talking about change and ready to create it.

Her debut book—and first work outside her professional field—*Your Second Prime: Does Aging Suck, or Do We Suck at Aging?* delivers a bold and personal rethinking of what it means to age in modern society. Drawing on epigenetics, behavioral science, and a personal health scare that turned her assumptions inside out, the book offers both practical guidance and a philosophical challenge: Why have we accepted decline as inevitable, and what becomes possible when we stop?

Through her podcast and public speaking, Gretchen cuts through wellness-industry noise to reconnect people with what truly matters: their health, their purpose, and their capacity to begin again—at any age.

Gretchen believes we've spent too long chasing answers to the wrong questions—especially about aging. Her work invites a shift from certainty to curiosity, from assumptions to awareness. Because the future isn't something we figure out—it's something we learn to see differently.